A NEW ENGLAND COUNTRY VETERINARIAN

MEMORIES AND MUSINGS

A NEW ENGLAND COUNTRY VETERINARIAN

MEMORIES AND MUSINGS

TERRY M. MILLS, DVM

Copyright © 2004 by TERRY M. MILLS, DVM

All rights reserved.

No part of this book may be reproduced, stored in a retrieval system, or transmitted by any means, electronic, mechanical, photocopying, recording, or otherwise, without written permission from the author.

ISBN: 1-58721-777-5 (paperback)

Illustrations by
Angela Wessling Marinelli
and her sister Lauren Wessling.

This book is printed on acid free paper.

1stBooks – rev. 07/26/04

This book is dedicated to my three daughters, Carolyn Mills-Meyer, Nancy DiGregorio and Joan Gray, whose talents with horses nudged me into the equine phase of my general practice.

INTRODUCTION

This book is a collection of what I like to call 'Vignettes' in the days of a New England country veterinarian. They touch on personal experiences, observations and opinions generated during over 50 years of association with the profession.

I hope it will be found interesting to those who may entertain a certain curiosity about such a life style.

I did my graduate work at Middlesex Veterinary College, Waltham, Mass., graduating with its first class in 1942. After which, with the exception of time out for service in WW II, I have been a solo General Practitioner.

Middlesex was not destined to last long and came to a halt in the late 40's when it became Brandies University. We were then left without an alma mater until recently when both Brandies and Tufts School of Veterinary Medicine granted us honorary graduate status. This was in recognition of the commendable service we have given to the profession for over 50 years.

PREFACE

There was a compelling drive in me to relate the thoughts and episodes that are put together in this little book. In trying to analyze the reasons for this obsession, I have decided them to be that - I enjoyed doing it, and of course I hoped some would enjoy reading it. But there is perhaps a more substantial reason for this obsession. It's about the country type vet who seems to be slowly disappearing from the scene. The vet I speak of perhaps had a small hospital for pets, but he also treated the local cattle, horses, pigs, sheep or practically any species that needed help. He did this essentially alone. The Teaching Universities were helpful but often far away. This life style embodied a very rugged, resourceful, all purpose individual. He worked hard, and was often exposed to the weather. He knew most of his clients, he lived long but never became rich. His wife was assistant and bookkeeper, his children were often volunteered for kennel work and company on the road. He sometimes worked on the barter system. This type of guy is not being replaced by the next generation. The inexorable tendency now is to specialize into large or small animals or group practices often with their own internal specialists. The hospitals are often elaborate copies of human hospitals. This all results in therapies beyond the reach of many traditional methods and often beyond the reach of what the low income owner can pay.

So what has all this to do with my compulsion to scribble all these stories down? It must be that I just don't want us to pass without being noticed.

If there is any resemblance to real people in these pages, it is probably true. I meant no harm. I loved you all.

TABLE OF CONTENTS

John's Colicky Mare 1
Mobile Home Dog 3
Chicken Graffiti 5
Milk Fever 7
Henry's Late Mare 9
Chicken Leg 11
Shattered Contentment 13
Back To The Drawing Board 15
Colorful Family Of Color 17
Double Trouble 19
Pinto In The Pasture 21
Human Animal Bonding 23
Dog Bites And Rabies 25
Common Sense 29
Adverse Reactions 31
Porcupine Quills 33
Gertie 37
New Anesthesia 39
Ellen's Virgin Poodle 41
X-Rays In The Field 43
Microcosm 45
Beer And Ether Don't Mix 47
Retreat Reflex 49
Ronnie's Perfect Horse 51
Long Tooth 55
Most Favorite Animals 57
The Real News 59
Cows Are Stupid 61
Purchase Exams 65
Ketosis – Reducing Diet 69
Oops Or Ah Ha S 71
Loose Horse Tragedy 73
Ike The Runaway Horse 75
Oh Boy It's Stuck 79
Compassion 81

Horse Laugh	83
Population Explosion	85
You Killed My Cat	87
Decision To Euthanize	89
What Goes On Here	91
19th Century Preferred	95
Breech	97
Preventive Medicine	101
All In A Day's Work	103
Proud Of His Scars	105
Saddle Bag Call	109
Fred's Old Wooden Barn	111
Expect The Unexpected	113
These Are Your Pups	117
Sit On The Head	119
Big Hearted Souls - Small Minded Souls	123
Horse Show Vet	127
John Long Polish Name	131
Feeling Guilty	133
Zoonosis	135
Who Is Your Vet	137
Misguided Good Intentions	139
Sneak Attack	141
I'll Take Him	143
Distemper	145
The Eye Of The Horse	147
Riding Lessons	151
Dogs For Health	153
Do Animals Think	155
Aging A Horse	159
Bad Times – Good Times	161
Heroics	163
Thunder Struck	165
Decapitation	167
No Retirement	169
The Potent Geldings	171
When To Retire	173
Vignettes	175

Don't Touch Me	179
Emotions And Colic	181
May You Have A Long Life	183
Swamp Fever	185
Vengeful Skunk	189
Animal Rights	191
Up To Date Rabies	197
Torsion Of The Uterus	199
Speedy Dachshund	201
But Doc -	203
Grandparents	205
Hot Tip	207
It Was Worth It	209
Insurance Salesman	211
In Support Of General Practice	213
Winnie	215
Attitude	221
Stay Of Execution	223
It All Washes Off	227
Casey Is Missing	229
Great Blue Heron	231
Part Of The Solution	233
Peter's Coast Guard Recruit	235
Lady Bug	237
At The Farmer's Fair	239
Contentment	243
Compassion Vs Cash	245

JOHN'S COLICKY MARE

John delivered his milk daily to the Farmer's Co-op by team. He was in his 70's and the old ways suited him just fine. He also had a sense of humor and was a good observer on life. He was a good man to know.

The Farmers' Co-op was put together by a local group of dairymen to process their milk. It was more efficient than each one trying to pasteurize, homogenize and bottle his own product. It functioned well until one by one the family farms disappeared.

John had little use for modern farming. No need to drive a truck, he had his beloved team. No need for milking machines, he milked by hand. From time to time I was called to see his cows. I always allowed time for chatting with him and usually picked up a bit of old time wisdom. It was one of the joys of a country practice.

5 AM - milking time for John. This morning he hurried back to the house to make a phone call. "Doc, my mare is sick, she can't make her water." "Tell me what she's doing." I said. "She's squatting down, looking at her side, pawing the floor and she won't eat." "John," I said, "She has colic, not a urine stoppage." I told him how to use my favorite home colic remedy consisting of baking soda, ginger, whiskey and hot water, and to call me back if she wasn't better. "She's trying to make water, Doc, you'd better check her out!" John was very concerned about his mare. The sooner colic is treated the better, so - on with the boots and the headlights.

The mare was obviously in pain just as John had said. I made a diagnosis of colic and gave the proper medicine for it. She failed to respond. The pelvic exam was next. With my long sleeve on and lubricated I started to exam the intestines expecting to find where the cause of the colic was. As my hand passed over the pelvic rim I felt an egg shaped object that appeared to be lodged in the neck of the urinary bladder. The bladder was over filled. "Could it be that John was right and I was wrong?" The mare resented pressure on her bladder and threatened to kick me. Drawing on courage that I didn't know I had, I forced what was apparently a bladder stone through the urethra into the vagina and hence into the outside world. It was followed by release of a great amount of urine, a sigh of relief from the mare, and a smug look on John's ugly face. "She'll feel fine now," I said, "she couldn't urinate!" John never indulged in the urge to say, "I told you so," for which I was duly grateful. He was just too happy to be able to drive his team to town that morning.

9 AM - Back on the road and realizing that most of whatever I knew was preceded by a mistake. This taught me to listen very closely to the client.

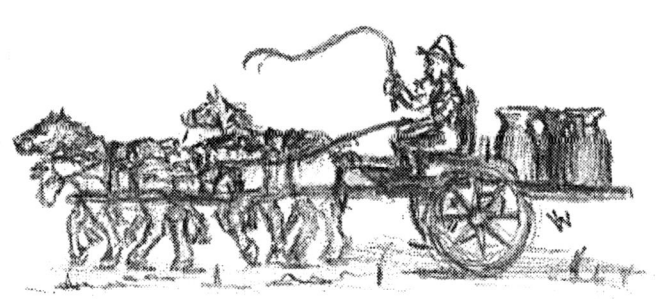

MOBILE HOME DOG

An oversized mobile home parked in the road, it was too big to fit in my parking lot. They came in with a little Terrier type dog. They said they lived in the mobile home. I was fascinated with their life style so I engaged them in conversation, as I am prone to do with interesting people. Seems they traveled year round in their mobile home following the seasons. The foundation of their house was their wheels, their front walk was an Interstate Highway, their yard was any trailer park. He had a little work shop in the rear of the mobile home where he used tin cans to make replicas of the 'Tin Man' from the 'Wizard of Oz'. They were cute, I bought one and my wife loved it. They had adopted the little dog from a pound in Georgia. Heading north they fell in love with her, but she coughed and scratched a lot and she didn't smell good. Seeing my Veterinary sign they decided to seek help for their new dog. I examined her and noted the following conditions:

Sarcoptic mange
Fleas
Ear Mites
Hook Worms
Whip Worms
Heart Worms
Pregnancy - third trimester

A very healthy little dog with a parade of treatable conditions.

The owners stayed in town until all problems were resolved, including a late pregnancy spay. Then they hit the road again.

Since that time they have faithfully arranged their travel schedule to park in the road in front for the little dog's annual check up. She remains in good health and seems to enjoy the fantastic good fortune that abruptly changed her life style from a dog pound to a nomadic home on wheels.

CHICKEN GRAFFITI

One of my hobbies is raising Banty Chickens. They lower my blood pressure, like watching gold fish. I also have a client who raises chickens for a hobby. Whenever he brings his old Doberman in for adjustments, chicken talk happens before he leaves. The time came for the yearly check up on his dog. While making the appointment he mentioned that one of his chickens was losing it's feathers and the others were picking at it. I suggested that he put the chicken in a sky kennel and bring it along with the dog. That didn't seem too extraordinary to me or to my client but to his daughter it was hilarious and she saw a chance to poke some fun at her father. She took the sky kennel that was to be used for transporting the chicken and spent the evening decorating it with graffiti. When the sky kennel made it to my office, I was so amused at her work that I thought it should be shared.

She had plastered this all over the chicken sky kennel -

To the Vet's or bust.
No fowl language.
Stay out of hot water.
Hen Again's Ale
My owner spent his nest egg on my eggucation.
Birds of (no) feather - well let's just say don't flock together.
Eat pork
My boss pays me chicken feed
I'm so eggcited
Support your local fowls.
Hens off.

My client was slightly apologetic at first but soon realized how much we enjoyed it. I couldn't decide what was wrong with the chicken, so I used my favorite treatment - keep 'em alive until they get better.

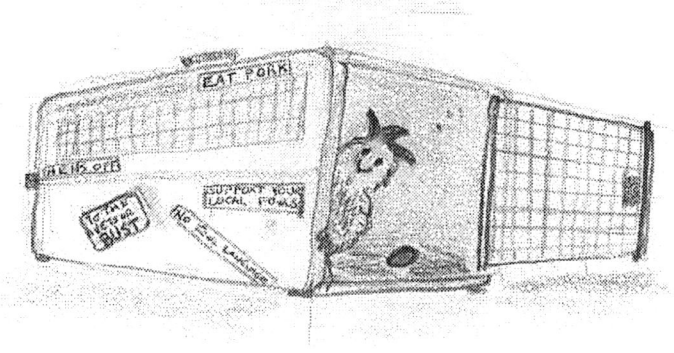

MILK FEVER

In the early days of World War II while starting an internship with a general practitioner, I learned what it was like when every case was a first case. No place for the faint of heart. My boss was away for the weekend. I was left in charge.

"Doc, my cow is down, barely breathing, calved two days ago. Can you come?" Milk Fever! Milk Fever is a common problem in dairy cows. It is a misnomer. It has nothing to do with fever. It is caused by low blood calcium. The increased demand for calcium due to calving and milk production fails to be replaced in the blood from other sources. Calcium is a necessary component for the transformation of nerve stimulae into muscle action. Depletion of this results in the paresis of Milk Fever. The treatment of Milk Fever is replacement of the blood calcium and perhaps is one of the most dramatic in veterinary medicine. Coma and paralysis is often reversed before one's eyes.

Anticipating the problem, I grabbed the calcium-gluconate and intravenous equipment and headed out with the first case jitters. The cow's ears were down, her tail was down, her eyelids were down, her pulse was down, her temperature was down, her breathing was down, she was down out and starting to bloat. And I was scared. Paralyzed fore stomachs in a cow quickly bloat because of the fermentation going on. Constant burping is part of their life style. I handed the bottle of calcium to the owner, secured her head to one side and hit the Jugular vein on the third try. About half of the bottle was administered with no visible results. The owner was wishing that his regular vet was there and so was I.

Suddenly her ears flapped and her tail twitched. Next she came up on to her brisket, burped a mighty burp, and started chewing her cud. She looked around like - "What's all the fuss about?" After a bit, we helped her up and I went back feeling quite heroic.

Two hours later the phone woke me -- "Doc she's down again." Wondering what I had done wrong, I got out of bed and repeated the treatment. This time she stayed up. I slept good the rest of the short night.

Some years later, after 2 years in the service, married and with a baby, I had another milk fever case that sticks in my memory.

Archie lived next door. He was an elderly retired carpenter who was anxious for any diversion. He loved to ride with me on my afternoon farm calls. I looked foreword to his company. His tales broke the monotony on the ride between calls. This case was unusual in that the cow had collapsed in a narrow entry way to the barn, completely blocking the way of the other cows anxious to get in for the night milking. The cows were hungry and their udders were full and uncomfortable. Archie was not used to a farm environment. He was of the urban sort who thought milk just came in bottles. His amazement at the sight of a cow collapsed in a walk way causing a cow traffic jam, was matched only by the sight of her recovery and return to her stanchion.

On the return trip Archie was complimenting me on my apparent miracle act, while I was thinking how the real credit should go to the guys who discovered the cause of and treatment for the disease. But the compliments were sweet so I let him continue. It broke the monotony.

HENRY'S LATE MARE

Henry raised, trained and showed Appaloosas. He was a natural horseman who had good control of his horses, he understood them and they trusted him. He eventually became a respected horse show judge. It was always a pleasure to travel the twenty miles to administer to his horses.

In those days my small animal work was done in the morning and the afternoon saw me out with the horses. Late afternoon was not popular with dairymen because it was the all important milking time. Most horsemen however welcomed the late afternoon time because they had day jobs. This meant that my assistant daughter and I seldom had an evening meal - except at Henry's. It was traditional with Henry and Flo to corral us into their kitchen after the work was done for a great meal. They were good friends.

There came a time when Henry had a valuable mare late in pregnancy. He called me every day from day 350 of the pregnancy on. "Why doesn't she foal. Is she all right?" I assured him every day that she was fine and for him to be patient. Day 365 came, still no foal. At this point even I became concerned. I happened to be working in the area late one day. Instead of going home I decided to stop in at Henry's to see for myself what was going on. It was a fortunate decision. Henry was glad to see me. He was now distraught and bleary eyed from keeping a night watch on his tardy mare. "Henry", I said, "Why don't you let me examine the mare? If she meets three criterions I can induce her, then we can be with her when she foals and you can get a night's sleep. The three criterions were, one - at least 350 days of pregnancy; two - milk in her udder; and three - a relaxed cervix. She met all three. Henry said, "Let's go for it." We bandaged her tail, washed her, and I injected the necessary medicine. Then we left her alone to avoid any distractions. Twenty minutes later she was lying down and in labor. At this point I risked delaying the birthing process and got her up for an exam to be sure the foal was properly positioned. Any mal-position is best corrected before the foal is squeezed into the birth canal. The position was fine. We disappeared again so the parturition process could restart. Ten minutes later we found her down again and twenty minutes after that two feet were presented to the outside world. I checked again to be sure the head was not turned back. Then I asked Henry if he wanted to help with the delivery by applying traction to the legs as the mare contracted. He was more than eager to get into the act and was immediately on the stall floor helping to deliver his foal. The foal was delivered in good health. The only mishap was Henry lost his cap as the foal slithered out. It was eventually recovered soiled with all sorts of birthing fluids and bedding. We left the umbilical chord intact to the placenta until the foal attempted to rise to permit infusion of any remaining blood into the foal. Within an hour the foal struggled to it's feet and shortly after found the source of first milk (colostrm). We waited patiently for it to pass its first bowel movement (meconium). Then having met the three hurdles of standing, drinking and passing meconium it was launched on a successful foalhood. Henry cherished the uncleaned cap for a long time afterwards.

    In due time the mare probably would have foaled on her own, but induction was indicated at this point and it has its advantages. It allows help to be there if needed and it frees the owner from the agony of sleepless nights. Hours of night watching can be rewarded by the mare doing her thing when one takes a half hour nap or makes a dash to the toilet.
    The long ride home that night gave me a chance to dwell on some of the rewards of a country practice that can often outweigh the monetary rewards.

CHICKEN LEG

They made good use of my being a general practitioner. At various times I treated their dogs, cats, goats, horses and pot bellied pig, and, oh yes, a chicken. Their four year old daughter had a pet chicken that was careless around the horses and suffered a broken leg thereby. I put a splint on the leg and after a few weeks the chicken was able to throw away its crutches.

One cold night I was called to treat their two year old colt with colic. We worked a long time into the night with the case and eventually resolved it. I was proud of the result.

A National Magazine called for contributions to a contest to name one's favorite Country Vet and why he or she was picked. Joan, the lady of this household decided to enter my name in the contest. She took a flattering picture of me with my Boxer and sent in her competition, along with an explanation of why she picked me. I was one of the winners and my picture was printed along with why I was her favorite country vet. The reason I am relating all this is because of her extraordinary reason for picking me. I expected to be cited for my many successful resolutions of their animal health problems, especially the mid-nite horse colic. No way! I made a National Magazine because I fixed the leg of her daughter's pet chicken. This has been a source of amusement for me and others.

I am in fact grateful for Joan's effort because it resulted in my hearing from several friends around the country that I had lost contact with. And considering the appreciation I got from her little daughter, I am as proud of the chicken leg as any of the rest.

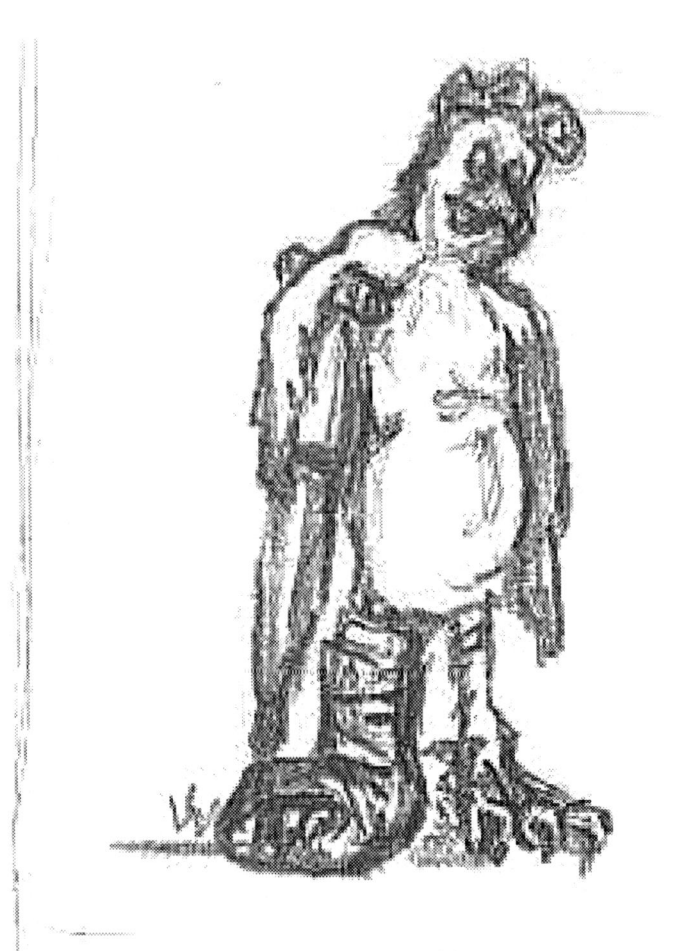

SHATTERED CONTENTMENT

There is something comforting about the lighted windows of a dairy barn in the pre-dawn darkness. The cows are fed and contented, the gutters are cleaned and the farmer is doing the morning milking.

On this pre-dawn morning the contentment was shattered. The farmer had found a cow exhausted from labor with no sign of relief. It was cold, snowy and dark but the lighted windows of the barn cheered me as I approached it. I knew it would be warm with animal heat inside.

The cow was in hard labor with nothing to show for her efforts. I tied her tail out of the way, cleaned the area and put on a shoulder length sleeve. The vaginal exam caused my arm to twist to the right. Diagnosis - torsion (twist) of the uterus. The calf had flipped over in late pregnancy causing a 180 degree twist of the uterus and consequent narrowing of the birth canal, making presentation of the fetus impossible. Back to the van for proper instruments - a long steel rod with a ring at both ends and two obstetrical chains. I squeezed my arm through a tight cervix that would normally have been relaxed, guiding a chain to make a loop around a front ankle. The rod was then introduced and the chain fed through the ring and around the other ankle and back through the ring, then out to be secured to the ring at the other end of the rod. This had the effect of binding the feet to the ring so that when the rod was rotated it produced an anti torsion force on the calf. The resistance was severe, but following an on and off anti rotation effort there was a pronounced movement of the calf indicating it's return to a normal position. There was a sigh of relief from the owner, the vet and the cow. Usually at this point the vet can put away his instruments and await a normal delivery, which was the case on this winter morning. We relaxed, discussed the weather and the price of milk and when the cow laid down for delivery she needed very little help from us. The day would be long, but it started good and nothing after that would be apt to spoil it.

On the way back I stopped for breakfast and got to thinking about the difference between dairy and horse veterinary work. Dairy barns provide a warm place to work in the winter and the milk room is a good place to clean up with warm water. Horse stables are cold and seldom have the luxury of warm water. Dairymen are in business and seldom have time for idle conversation other than the weather and the various difficulties of farming. Companion horses, on the other hand are usually the owner's hobby which means that we always allow time for a coffee break to talk about our horsey experiences.

BACK TO THE DRAWING BOARD

My wife as an observer of the horse scene has made the comment that the species horse should be sent back to the drawing board. She was referring to the slender legs which she considers entirely inadequate to support the massive body, and she thinks the guts that have all nite colics need redesigning She's right, horses are prone to many kinds of lamnesses and belly aches.

One of the most dramatic types of lameness occurs when a rear leg suddenly becomes as stiff as a two-by-four. It actually can be moved only from the hip. It comes on suddenly and occasioally corrects itself just as suddenly. If it persists, it is clearly an emergency.

As the stifle (knee) is bent the patella (knee cap) normally glides up and down in a groove on the end of the femur. The Patella is attached to the lower bone (tibea) by three ligaments - medial, middle and lateral. In this case the patella apparently slips up a bit too high allowing the medial and middle ligaments to lock over a protuberance on the end of the femur. This locking action prevents the stifle and the hock from bending. The condition is dramatic. The treatment is equally dramatic. Many lamenesses are ill defined, prolonged and recurring. Not this one. A surgical procedure involving dividing of the medial patellar ligament brings immediate relief. The after affects are minimal.

My first case went like this. On a Sunday afternoon my wife called me in from repairing fences and sent me post-haste to a good client who was panicked because her Morgan mare suddenly could not straighten a rear leg. She said it was just dragging behind her. I sensed what the trouble was and my anxiety mounted. I knew what the surgical procedure was, but had never done it. I gathered up a neighborhood boy who was always more than eager to ride with me. At the scene we tried to relieve the condition by pulling the leg foreward. This failed, so I announced that I would have to do the surgery. As I was gathering my instruments, the boy appeared at the truck and whispered, "Have you ever done this before?" He was obviously shaken and completely lacking confidence in me. This of course was exactly what I didn't need at this point. Drawing on courage that was there only because there was no other choice, I did the surgery and the mare walked normally back into her stall. On the return trip the boy apologized for his lack of confidence. I was so relieved at the outcome that I easily forgave him. The fence waited a week to be repaired.

There are many reasons for horses being prone to colic. One has more to do with management than the horse. It involves the way the horses are fed. Horses are naturally grazers which means that they eat small amounts more or less continually during day light hours. Domesticated horses are often fed grain on an empty stomach and hay only two or three times a day. This results in the stomach being empty for hours which is not normal and may lead to various forms of trouble. Well managed stables have fewer cases of colic than poorly managed ones.

Obviously we cannot send the horse back to the drawing board to change his guts that have evolved over thousands of years and have contributed to his survival as a species in the face of predation and Ice Ages. Any changing must be done by us. We must follow as closely as possible to the horse's natural instinctive habits.

COLORFUL FAMILY OF COLOR

A colorful family of color boarded a horse with us for a time. They had a fine big Thoroughbred Hunter and a son who showed ability in riding and horsemanship. The boy represented a minority on two fronts. He was a black and he was a boy. Most horse show participants are girls for some unknown reason. This failed to deter him. But this little story; is about his father, the colorful part of the family. He had a sense of humor that often came as a surprise.

For instance -He looked at my daughter after she had returned from a Florida visit and said, "You didn't get much tan, you don't even qualify to ride in the back of the bus." At another time "Doc you did a great job on my horse, thank you very very much." I of course replied with false modesty. Then he said, "Now that will take care of the bill." That remark as I recall did take care of some of the bill. Another time at a horse show food stand he asked his son if he wanted some fried chicken. The son declined. "What," he said, "who ever heard of a Nigger that don't want fried chicken!" As I said, this family was colorful, but more importantly they discouraged any thought of discrimination with their up-beat attitude and their humor that often poked fun at themselves.

DOUBLE TROUBLE

Lounging at home in front of the fire, slippers on, half asleep; the phone rings. "Doc I have a problem, Don is away and our mare is terrible, she has colic and she's having trouble breathing." I recognized Jane's voice and I remembered that the mare was subject to asthmatic attacks. "What can I do?" she said hysterically. This meant to me-"Get your butt down here." I knew better than to delay. Slippers off, boots and headlights on.

Jane and Don were Morgan people. We competed with them at horse shows and frequently came together as friends. It was always a pleasure to travel the 25 miles to treat their animals then eat and talk at their table after the work was done. They were good friends.

I thought of this on the hurried drive down there and hoped that I could save the horse and the friendship. Colic always has the chance of fatality. Colic plus asthma at the same time was a real challenge.

The mare was indeed in trouble. She was in pain, her nostrils were dilated, she made great heaving efforts to breathe and she was covered with white frothy sweat. She had a severe attack of asthma! Her pulse was elevated, her membranes were pale, there was no rumbling in her belly. She was making violent efforts to lie down. She had severe colic! The mare was being held up by two strong men who were nearly exhausted. A really desperate scene.

My first move was to relieve her pain and fear with a tranquilizer. Then a catheter was introduced into her jugular vein to give medications and fluids for maintaining blood pressure. Next a tube was passed through her nose into her stomach. This was to relieve accumulated gas and provide a way to give medicine for the colic. The mare's difficulty with breathing prevented us from walking her, which is often done with colic cases.

There we struggled for some time, trying to maintain the various portals into the mare's body, trying to keep her on her feet, encouraging the guys who were holding her up, expecting the worst and hoping for the best.

After about an hour of struggling with the desperate situation we noticed that her nostrils were a bit less dilated, her pulse had leveled off and her legs were not folding under her as often. We looked at each other with expressions that said, "Maybe!"

We were in the kitchen with coffee and donuts. The mare was eating hay, calmed down, dried off and acting very much as though, "What's all the fuss about?" I was getting great praise for my expertise, my late at night devotion to duty etc. etc. and was happily accepting all the accolades when a sobering thought hit me. "Wasn't I just a messenger in all this?" If it is said, "Don't kill the messenger," then why should we praise the messenger? The real heroes were the clinical pioneers who developed the medicines and techniques making all this possible. I drove home happy about the results with the horse and the preserved friendship but with the whole picture put into proper perspective.

PINTO IN THE PASTURE

Returning from delivering health care to dairy cows late one winter afternoon, I was surprised to see a car on the opposite side of our stone fence resting serenely in the pasture. This was unusual so I investigated. The driver was a young woman. It seems she had lost control of her car on some ice and they vaulted over the fence to land where I found them, apparently both unharmed. In fact she seemed quite pleased with herself. I was curious about one thing so I asked the gal, "Just between us, how fast does one have to go in order to do a thing like that." I never got an answer because a policeman had arrived on the scene and she wasn't about to incriminate herself. By that time a small crowd of sightseers had gathered. I decided that it was time to think about removing the jumping car from our land and was eager to divert some of the attention to myself, after all it was my pasture that her car was sitting in. So I hurried off to get my tractor, intending to attach a chain and pull her out to the road. It was winter, as I said, and the old John Deere's 6 volt battery was too weak to start it, thereby frustrating my good intentions. About that time I heard a loud roar. It was made by the car crawling up the bank with my daughter driving and several guys pushing. That rained on my parade and my role as a hero was ruined. As the car went by I noticed that it was a Pinto, so I decided to talk business with the gal. After things calmed down I said to her "If you want to board your horse in our pasture it's negotiable, but the fact that he jumps fences may be a problem." She didn't think it was as funny as I did, and she left. I went back to the tractor and kicked the left rear tire.

HUMAN ANIMAL BONDING

Bonding between animal and owner is an acknowledged fact in the American way of life. It may be that the further we advance into a sophisticated technical artificial way of life the more we find a need for this bonding. Perhaps it is in response to an unconscious need to preserve our primordial interdependence with other species? Whatever the cause, it is a forceful aspect in our lives and brings comfort to many.

Companion animal veterinarians work entirely within this bonding mind set and need to work in a social-economic system that provides opportunity for discretionary spending on this bonding emotion. As a matter of fact if this animal- man bond were non existent, so would be the companion animal vet.
Veterinary Medicine would be confined to food producing animals and control of zoonotic diseases such as TB, Rabies, and others.
(Zoonotic diseases are those contagious from animals to man).
I suspect that without this companion animal love affair and the companion animal vets the world would go on quite nicely, although somewhat mal-adjusted and much less happy. It might be well if from time to time companion vets tasted a little humble pie and paused to realize that we are dependent on an economic system that provides above maintenance spending and on an emotion that in some societies does not exist.

Examples of bonding are everywhere, our family is no exception. It is said that a man has one real good dog in his life time. I have had three; a Mongrel, a Doberman Pinscher and a Brittany Spaniel. With the death of a pet most bonding runs a normal course. The pet is grieved adequately, then life goes on. There are extremes, however. Let me tell of a few.

This one involves a photograph. These interesting people let their diabetic dog linger long after good sense would dictate that they should let him slip away. When he finally died they appeared at my office with a picture of their deceased dog for me to admire. Not knowing how to respond to this, I commiserated with them and suggested that they really shouldn't keep the picture.

Another incident involves bonding after the death of the owner. In fact this may represent an example of animal-human bonding contributing to human-human bonding. It went like this. The dog was a beautiful Sheltie (Shetland Sheep Dog), fortunate enough to be owned by a lovely devoted lady who was also at this time very ill. This lovely lady had a sister who wanted to help out all she could. The Sheltie's owner was in the hospital, not expected to live. Her sister was determined that the owner should see her Sheltie dog to help in the cure or at least to bring comfort. Of course dogs were not allowed in the hospital, so she decided to circumvent the rules.

She did this by having herself pushed into the hospital in a wheel chair with the dog on her lap covered by a blanket. The reunion was a success and brought comfort to the owner who shortly passed away. After her death the little Sheltie continued looking for her owner to the point of distraction. The still loyal sister took things into her own hands again. In order to convince the dog of it's owner's death she carried him into the funeral parlor to allow the dog to see for himself that his owner was deceased. After this the dog understood that his owner was gone, mourned for awhile and went on with his life.

It is not my purpose to ridicule these fine people. The bond with their pets was perhaps extreme, but it would be a dull world without unique people.

DOG BITES AND RABIES

Whether out of meaness or fear, it hurts to be bitten by a dog. Veterinarians view it as an occupational hazard and pay little regard to it. A quick wash and a dab of iodine has kept me alive for years. Most biters are of the fear type, or the 'stay away from me' ones. These are usually represented by very small dogs or those who were not properly socialized as young puppies. The mean type are the 'don't touch me' ones. Topping the list of the mean type in our opinion are Chows and Rotweillers. Chows have a 'don't touch me' attitude. They are hard to control because of a heavy coat of hair on a thick neck. Rotweillers can be friendly but their threshold of patience with any sort of medical handling is short and their response can be quick and dangerous. Of course there are exceptions as with any rule, and some of the trouble can be with the owner's lack of control. Occasionally there are 'attack biters', which are indeed a 'dog' of another color, (stay tuned). In this case the dog advances aggressively with intent to knock down and do major damage.

Topping the list of stoic, forgiving patients are Poodles and surprisingly, Doberman Pinschers. Dobermans are greatly maligned by the television media. They are used only when there is need for some ferocious white teeth. Our family had Dobermans in the home and on the farm for thirty years. Their high profile in our yard supported by their television image helped protect us from break-ins during all that time. On the other hand there was never any blood shed and our insurance man still talked to us.

Boxers are also good patients, however, as I mentioned, there are exceptions. Here is one of them. We were boarding a Boxer with instructions to up-date him. We had had him a few days with no trouble. He was on the ward floor in preparation for the exam. I turned my back for some equipment when I heard a scuffle. I wheeled around to see him backing my assistant into the wall, jumping at her throat. I pulled him off and secured him in a kennel. The assistant was treated for a deep bite wound on her wrist. This was an 'attack biter'.

When the owner came for his dog I told him exactly what had happened. I was hoping he wouldn't take a defensive attitude toward his dog, but at the same time felt that he should know what his dog was capable of doing. Apparently the dog had an unprovoked sense of <u>rage</u>, which should be differentiated from <u>fear</u>. The owner's response was wise and impressive. He said, "Keep the dog for the necessary quarantine, then put him to sleep." He thanked me for my candor, paid me in advance and left looking sad. Attack bites are fortunately rare, but bites hurt no matter what the reason.

This may be a good time to talk about Rabies. Rabies is caused by a virus that attacks nerve tissue, producing gradual paralysis starting usually in the throat region. This makes swallowing difficult and is why it is called 'hydrophobia' (fear of water). All warm blooded animals are susceptible. Human exposure is usually from dogs or bats and currently raccoons, however it can be spread by any animal in the acute stage of the disease. It is transmitted by a bite wound or rarely a scratch. It is not spread by aerosol or contact as in a cold. Rabies vaccine is very effective and has been important in controlling the disease in dogs and humans. It is also given as a precautionary measure to horses and ferrets and others. The virus is in the saliva of a dog in the acute stage of rabies, making the transmission by a bite highly probable. The afflicted dog will die within ten days. This is why there is a mandatory quarantine of ten days for the dog guilty of biting. If he outlives the ten days, he did not have rabies and the person bitten will not get the disease. If he succumbs during the quarantine period his brain is tested for the disease and if positive the person bitten is vaccinated against the disease. There is a relatively long incubation period with Rabies (time from exposure to the appearance of symptoms.) This is fortunate because it allows time for the series of preventative vaccines to become effective in the exposed human.

Perhaps you can see from this that Veterinary medicine is by no means concerned with just animals. It very often concerns itself with humans, their joys, sorrows and their difficult decisions. Veterinarians serve inclusively from fertility doctors to undertakers, with some barbering in between. The variety is part of the charm of the profession.

COMMON SENSE

As I lay on my back for an X-Ray of my knee that had been impacted by the hoof of an unreasonable horse, the technician asked me what kind of a doctor I was. When I said that I was a Veterinarian she perked up her ears and told me about her cats. Seems she had two 18 year old cats and she asked me what she should feed them. I replied, "My dear, it would be presumptuous of me to give advice to anyone who has kept her cats to 18 years of age. You have done well without my advice."

Then she started on how she had noticed a change in veterinarians lately. She said she felt the profession was tending to get out of control. Her old vet had retired. In self defense she had told her new young vet that all she wanted with her cats' annual check up was to do just the obvious and to please avoid extremes in testing and treating the inevitable progress of old age.

Sensing what she was trying to say, I tried to explain. I pointed out that recent graduates had been taught all the latest approaches to medical problems so were naturally eager to apply them. Not having the advantage of years of experience they tend to rely on tests for a diagnosis instead of using tests to support a diagnosis. I call it the 'high tech high cost' approach to veterinary medicine. This is fine for many folks but it sometimes separates the common sense client from the common sense vet. The older 'common sense' vets are slowly folding their tents, to the regret of some and the satisfaction of others. Such is the way of all progress.

ADVERSE REACTIONS

Good luck is a help in any endeavor. Veterinary medicine is no exception. There are times when it happens and there are times when we wished it would happen. This is a little story about turning bad technique into good luck.

Somewhere in the 50's we were given a new class of drugs called tranquilizers. They became useful in many ways for man and beast. One use for the veterinarian was to calm a frightened horse or to ease the pain of colic. Equine colic is a serious threat as any horse owner knows. A phone call for colic is always treated as an emergency by the vet. He never knows whether he'll be back in an hour or be gone all night. The vet hopes for a quick cure but the possibility of surgery or death or both weighs on his mind. Any recovery from colic from whatever course of action is a great satisfaction to the vet, the owner and of course the horse.

It was a cold night in January. The pony had all the signs of painful colic. When I arrived the whole family and several neighbors were in the barn desperate to see some relief for their little friend. The patient was so painful that I decided to use the new tranquilizer immediately.

One caution with the new drug was that if it were given in an artery instead of a vein it might have the exact opposite effect from tranquilizing.

I administered the tranquilizer and the poor little creature immediately went into what could be described as an epileptic fit. He went down kicking and rolling, scattering pails, hay forks and onlookers. The whole group looked on in horror thinking I had killed their little friend. I was thinking along the same lines. NOT SO! After about three minutes of the violent reaction the pony suddenly got up, shook himself and started eating hay, a beautiful sign of recovery. Apparently the injection had inadvertently entered the carotid artery which lies just below the jugular vein. The resultant convulsion had undoubtedly shaken loose an impaction in the intestines, hence the relief. I regained my composure and seeing nothing to be gained by the truth, said, " That was a new treatment I only use in extreme cases." I don't know if they believed me but I do know that they never called me back. Anyhow the pony and all his friends were greatly relieved, and I used up some of my allotted good luck.

The subject of tranquilizers brings to mind another incident emphasizing the risks involved. This time it was a goat. I gave a small dose to a goat preparing it for dehorning.
Instead of becoming tranquilized it went into a deep coma.
Mid-night found the goat, the owner and me in her kitchen giving intravenous fluids and coffee to the slowly recovering goat.

Goat in the kitchen reminds me of another adverse reaction incident. A goat had an infection after giving birth (kidding), she was given a routine injection of penicillin. I left and an urgent call sent me back to the scene of the crime on the double. The penicillin had caused a reaction that put the goat into a coma. Mid night found the goat and the owner and me in the warmth of her kitchen giving fluids and stimulants to save the goat but not my reputation.

PORCUPINE QUILLS

A dog with Porcupine quills is always considered an emergency. They are painful and depending on the number can be dangerous. Painful or dangerous, it is not unusual for a dog to repeat his mistake more than once. It is also not unusual for an evening at home to be interrupted by a frantic call from the owner of a dog with a face full of quills. They seem to come in bunches. It is hard for me to believe that wild predators make that mistake more than once. Perhaps our domesticated dogs have a primordial urge to again be the great hunter, and the slow moving Porcies are easy prey. The only natural predator of the Porcies is the Fisher. It is claimed that this animal can overturn the Porcupine to get at it's defenseless under parts. When there are too many Porcupines in an area folks are apt to find their outside furniture chewed on, paint and all. To control their numbers Fishers are sometimes introduced into an area.

Porcupines have evolved a defensive mechanism unique to their species. The quills are modified hair and are loosely attached to the animal so they can exit easily. They have minute reverse direction barbs that make them very difficult to remove from the victim. All this, of course, discourages predators, except for Fishers and the dumber dogs. Contrary to popular belief, the Porcupine does not throw its quills. The tail is its first line of defense. By swinging it vigorously he is able to drive the quills into the nose of an approaching molester. Sometimes a dog gets so caught up with the hunt that he is covered with quills, which tells one that he survived the tail swing of the Porcie and attacked the body. Under anesthesia Veterinarians extract the quills, being careful not to break them off. Embedded quills are removed surgically.

The subject of quills brings to mind some of my rather interesting quill related experiences.-- After returning from the Service I was moving into my newly rented office when in came my first case, face full of quills. The only anesthesia available was ether. This had to be applied by a mask over the face, exactly where the quills were. This was awkward. We had to work fast between adequate and too light anesthesia. But we finished the job and I was able to continue moving in.

On another occasion, I was walking across my parking lot on my way home after a tiring day, when a van came smoking in on two wheels. "You got time for a quill job, Doc?" "I was just closing, but I guess I can do it", I said. The side door of the van opened. Out came a large Siberian Huskie, followed by a large Siberian Huskie, followed by large Siberian huskie, all loaded with quills.

He had fooled me, but I was committed, so with the owner's help we extracted hundreds of quills. The three Huskies went home half asleep dreaming happily of their great hunting success.

My wife's Doberman and my Boxer, behaving very badly, disappeared into the Adirondack woods near our camp just as we were leaving for the three and a half hour ride back home. We delayed our trip for a day, driving all over telling mountain folk of our dilemma. The dogs had Rabies tags with my office phone number on them. I pleaded with my wife that the best place to be was right by the phone. Anybody finding the dogs would be likely to phone my hospital and the people there would relay the info back to us. Reluctantly she agreed and reluctantly we had to leave for home in Massachusetts. This time I was right. We were home about an hour when the office called. The dogs had been found. One was tied up in a mountaineer's yard, and the Boxer was in a Veterinary Hospital with a face full of quills. I said, "Let them stay there over night, teach them a lesson." Not my wife, off she went on the return trip, to come back hours later with the two critters. Their story went like this. They were cruising through the woods when the Dobie spotted something moving behind a rock. He said to the Boxer, "Go see what that thing is." The Boxer did, and he and a Porcupine were introduced to each other. "He should have been more careful", the Dobie said. The Boxer limped into a neighbor's yard who kindly took him to a vet. I still say, the best place to be is close to a phone.

A little dog came in from a great hunting experience with so many quills in his face that it was turned white. I took a picture of it and put it on my bulletin board, labeling it 'Acupuncture'. I did it for a bit of humor but shortly had to take it down. Several people took it seriously, wondering why so many needles were necessary.

Porcie quills are what I like to call a 'grade one' problem. It's a painful emergency, the diagnosis is obvious, the treatment is straightforward and mechanical without much thinking called for. The problem and pain are relieved with one visit.

Nature has given animals a wonderful variety of defensive mechanisms. Some kick, some bite, some hide and some run. I recently read of what must be one of the most sophisticated defense systems in nature. The Monarch Butterfly, in it's larval stage feeds on Milk Weed which has a noxious substance affecting birds. This discourages birds from preying on the Monarchs. I stand in awe of such various intricacies of evolution guided by a Higher Intelligence.

GERTIE

Gertie was brought in to be put to sleep. She was a sweet little part Shepherd female, who had enjoyed about twelve summers. She had been found standing over her master who died suddenly in his chicken coop. There was no one in the family who wanted Gert, hence the sad mission to my office. I was given permission to find a home for her. This was unlikely with a twelve year old dog. We never got around to euthanizing her and she eventually gained freedom to roam around the hospital. Soon she began showing up during my office calls, and it became apparent that her unconcerned attitude was having a calming affect on the patients. We called her my canine receptionist. It was done in fun. The word reached a local reporter looking for an animal interest story. She took pictures and printed a cute Gertie story. This was picked up by other news papers and the little old lady dog eventually had wide media coverage as a canine receptionist. Her next move was to accompany me on my dairy calls, which leads to a humorous Gertie story. I'm not too sure this is proper for general consumption but I can't resist telling it.

After a cow calves her placenta is normally passed within a few minutes. 'Cleaning a cow' is the term used when the vet has to remove a retained placenta. This is an unpleasant task but gratifying in that the animal feels better and can now get on with her milk producing business. Gertie, probably responding to ancient hunting instincts, delighted in eating the discarded placentas. I of course discouraged this, but she was determined and smart. Back at the office on this particular day I was giving a job description to a new employee. Gertie, who at this time was finding the last stolen placenta more than her stomach could handle, started to divest herself of it. Vomiting while backing up she stretched out a long placenta covering half the length of the office floor. This was more than the new guy could stand. He went back to his job at McDonalds.

There are many jobs in Veterinary Medicine that could be considered distasteful. Listed among them are removing odorous retained placentas, rectal exams of cows and horses, cleaning up maggot infestations, etc. But it all washes off and is compensated for with a healing animal.

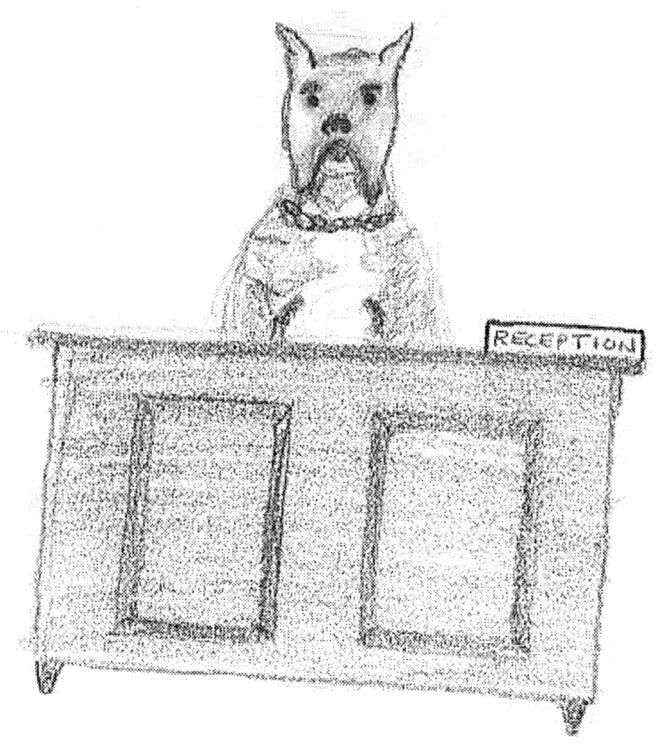

NEW ANESTHESIA

Whenever a new drug or procedure came along it was my habit to hold back for a year or so to let others learn the pit falls. You might say that I subscribed to the simple adage, "Be not the first by whom the new is tried, nor the last to lay the old aside". It was thus with intravenous anesthesia for field surgery in the horse. I deterred and watched. The loss of a patient through elective surgery is the worst case scenario for any doctor. Eventually it came my turn to adopt the new anesthesia.

A castrated horse is called a gelding. A gelding is a more contented and more useful horse than most stallions. The procedure has been done for hundreds of years. Up until the twentieth century it could hardly be called surgery. It was a brutal procedure that had no regard for pain and little for cleanliness. Since that time there has of course been many advancements in anesthesia and surgery.

It was on a Welsh Pony breeding farm. We sometimes had up to five colts to do at a time. This time there was only one. I decided to embark on the new procedure. A catheter was inserted into the jugular vein to administer the anesthesia. The pony went nicely to sleep. I prepped the area and started the surgery. There was only one problem. I was sacred stiff. Being occupied with the surgery and unfamiliar with the anesthesia, it was difficult for me to monitor the patient's breathing. Johnny the farm hand was my only assistant. I had always considered him to be a little slow, and he would soon prove it. As my anxiety increased and the sweat began to run down into my eyes, I cried out, "Johnny, how is he breathing?" Long pause in which my heart skipped a beat. "Johnny," I cried out again, "How is he breathing?" Finally after what seemed like an eternity, I heard Johnny mutter, "IN AND OUT, what do ya think!" His cool dry response relieved and composed me. The surgery continued to a successful end. Intravenous anesthesia became my habit and Johnny became dear to my heart.

ELLEN'S VIRGIN POODLE

Ellen was a very British woman with a very stylish Miniature Poodle. She and her Poodle were a reflection of each other. They fit the formula of owner-dog look alike. How she got to this country is rather interesting. Her future husband was in the Polish Navy when the Nazis attack on Poland brought about the British declaration of war. His unit escaped and joined the British Navy. He and Ellen were married in England and later emigrated to the U.S. This little Veterinary diversion is about Ellen and her Poodle.

Ellen's female Miniature Poodle was never let out alone (she said). On the phone this day she was very upset. As I listened to the description of her Poodle's discomforts, it became increasingly clear to me what her problem was. "Ellen", I said, "I think your dog is whelping". "Is what"? she shouted. "Having babies", I timidly replied. Her response was historic. "You are terribly mistaken", she screamed. "My poodle is never let out alone and if she was she'd never let that happen. I'm positive she's a virgin. You should apologize to her." Ellen's reaction was so explosive that I couldn't help but wonder if she had projected a life style into her dog that she herself might have missed.

Ellen was obviously greatly concerned, so I suggested she bring the little virgin right over for an exam. By the time she arrived she had two dogs with more to come. Fortunately her motherly instincts suppressed her fury and she became enthusiastic about her new family, lost virginity not withstanding.

How many times have I seen it happen? A dog in heat is carefully kept in for days. A child makes the mistake of leaving the door open and by evening the first cell divisions are taking place. Dogs have a relatively long heat period of about three weeks. When somebody asks me how long their dog will be in heat, I'm reluctant to answer because they often get upset with me, as though it was my fault.

X-RAYS IN THE FIELD

Taking X-Rays of a horse in the field is labor intensive and time consuming. The X-Ray machine is heavy and must be hauled to the scene along with cassettes, blocks for positioning the machine, and usually a system for positioning the patient's foot. The cassette and machine must be placed precisely. That's all the easy part. The real challenge is to get the patient to hold still during the exposure. Asking him to hold his breath or take a certain position is obviously futile. Many times the film may be spoiled by the horse moving just as the film is exposed. Assistants and owners must be protected from radiation exposure. The X-Ray machines are expensive and at risk of being dropped or kicked by the horse. I used to tell my assistant daughter, "If the horse moves, throw your body over the X-Ray machine." She took the remark in the manner in which it was given. If fact there were many times she snatched the machine out of harm's way.

All this having been done, the films must now be developed by the veterinarian or his staff. Finally the vet has to be the radiologist and interpret the films himself. Of course all this goes with the territory, but there are times we envy the human doctors who can avoid all the hassle.

MICROCOSM

A dog and his family create a symbiotic relationship. The family is good for the dog and the dog is good for the family, especially the children. A dog that is a playmate and guard for the children is nevertheless a lesser being that depends on his master for food and shelter and help in the time of need. A dog calls for discipline, reward, compassion and responsibility, each in its turn. What better way to help a child develop its character? A dog's life is like a microcosm of a human life. Youth, middle and old age are compressed into 15 or so years. There is a learning experience in this for children. Being with his friend through the challenges of advancing age and death can be a conditioning experience of real life for a child.

I have been with many concerned owners preparing for the death of their pet. Often they reach the decision to euthanize only to back off. My advice usually is to stay the course. The agonizing decision will only have to be made again in the near future.

BEER AND ETHER DON'T MIX

Beer and ether are a poor mix. Here's how I found out. After two years of interning, I finally started out on my own. I rented the bottom floor of a building which had a bar on the second floor. This was a satisfactory beginning arrangement - Until!

I was about ready to close up my little basement store front clinic one night when the phone rang and a very anxious voice said that his Beagle had been trying to whelp (give birth) all day. What was he to do? "She may need a Caesarian, bring her in, I'll wait for you," I said. My assistant had just left, I called him back. A Caesarian section was needed. Ether was the anesthetic of choice in those days. It worked fine but it had a penetrating odor. In fact it could penetrated right through to one's underwear and help bring on sleep at night. The surgery was about half done and there were some pups crying in a towel when there came a loud knock on the door. In came the bar tender complaining that the ether had gone through the floor and all his customers had left in disgust. I was embarrassed and sympathetic with the barkeep's problem but at the same time had trouble holding back a laugh which my assistant was completely unable to do. The barkeep was appeased when I agreed to use ether only in the mornings. There were few beer drinkers at that time of day, so a compromise was struck.

Shortly after that I was drafted into the service. It interrupted my struggling young practice, but solved a problem for the barkeep.

RETREAT REFLEX

"This time you are going to the emergency room." It was my assistant daughter speaking with conviction. She was shocked to see me flat on my back with blood running down my face.

Before this I had experienced a painful knee injury. The horse with his hind foot had bludgeoned my knee in the outward direction and hooked it for good measure on the return trip. Apparently he had resented the examination of a large Habronemia growth (caused by a type of fly larvae) on his penis. The owner had failed to mention that he had a mean streak. I ended up in the corner of the box stall on a pile of manure and my knee no longer worked properly. I had failed to seek medical help with the result that there was a slow recovery. This time I had no choice, she packed me into the truck, left all the equipment, and took off for the emergency room. It happened while we were working on a 4 month old colt. I foolishly made a quick move and lightning struck. It was the colt's front foot impacting my eye. There was no serious injury this time, just blood running down into my eye making it look terrible.

Working around animals one soon develops a quick retreat reflex. I have often said that the only reason I have all my appendages is because of this highly developed reflex. I have many scars, mostly from cats. Cats can put a number of holes into you without the courtesy of a warning. Other than the chance of infection they are generally not serious. I doubt any man's reflex can elude the unannounced strike of a cat.

An owner once had his face too close to the scene while I was conducting the exam. His dog threatened me, I reflexed out of the way and my fist hit the guy in the nose. There was some blood, but believe it or not I didn't get sued.

RONNIE'S PERFECT HORSE

Ronnie loved beautiful Quarter Horses. His habit was to buy one, show it for awhile to enhance its value then sell it so he could travel around looking for another. He'd often greet me with, "Hey Doc, you've got to stop over to see my new horse." I'd go and admire the horse, and the next time I stopped in it would be another horse. That was Ronny's style. He was a colorful guy and a good friend.

Tony was an experienced horseman, he had raised, trained and judged show horses most of his life. He went with Ronnie out West with the mission to bring back the best horse yet. Which is what they did.

"Hey Doc come see the new horse Tony and I brought back from the mid-west." I did and it was a beauty. "Tony and I looked this horse over from nose to tail, from the tip of his ears to soles of his feet. We longed him both ways and rode him at the walk, jog and lope. His wind and his eyes are good and he's sound of limb. This is the best one yet, he's perfect." I agreed that the horse indeed had exceptional conformation, and congratulated them on their ability to pick out the good ones.

Some time later while I was working a Sunday project on our farm, Ronny wheeled into the yard interrupting my day off. He jumped out of his truck, yelling, "Doc, my horse broke his jaw." "He what, how in the world did he do that?" "He fell and hit his nose on a curb. When he got up he was bleeding from the mouth. His upper jaw is broken."

When I examined the horse I was surprised to see that he had what is called a 'parrot mouth'. His upper incisors extended two inches beyond the lowers. When he fell he had hit his upper front teeth on a curb since they protruded beyond the lower ones that normally would have protected them. Apparently in going from the tip of his ears to soles of his feet they had omitted the mouth.

The upper jaw with the incisors were fractured and pushed upwards.

We anesthetized the gelding in his box stall, pushed the fractured jaw back in place and wired it securely to the first molars with stainless steel wire. The patient was muzzled and fed a liquid gruel for two weeks. Wounds around the head heal quickly. He made a complete recovery, and was returned to the status of Ronnie's perfect horse. But he wasn't a perfect horse. The lower arcade of teeth being set in a shorter jaw meant that the last lower molars and the first upper molars would fail to have opposing teeth to grind them down to proper levels. They would require rasping down by an equine dentist or a vet every year or so to maintain functional mastication. Since his perfect horse turned out to be not so perfect, I wasn't surprised when the next time I saw Ronnie he said, "Doc come see my new horse, she's a beauty. And this time we looked into her mouth!" The horse was indeed faultless. I admired the horse as usual while privately wondering if the new owner of Ronnie's previous less than perfect horse had looked into its mouth.

Another fractured jaw case was equally unusual and could serve here as a warning A stall door handle was made out of a horse shoe welded to a bar. The shoe was used as a handle to slide the bar back and forth into the latch. It worked good, but one night it was left sticking out in a horizontal position. The playful horse stuck his lower jaw through the horse shoe. You call imagine the rest. Both mandibles were broken behind the incisors in the space where the bit goes. This was treated by tapeing the mouth shut which brought the fractures into perfect alignment. The patient was fed a gruel through a stomach tube and muzzled to prevent him from using his jaw. The fracture healed quickly. He lost weight, and the tape left a bald spot on top of his nose, but it was a fair trade off. A small bar welded across the branch of the shoe would avoid this danger.

These are examples of how a country vet had to improvise in the days before University facilities and private large animal hospitals emerged on the scene. Things are better now, but some of the romance and challenges are gone.

LONG TOOTH

It is said that a horse is no better than his legs and as old as his teeth. Being herbivores, horses must spend a large part of their life eating. Their incisors in front are used for cutting off the forage, while their molars in back do the grinding. This calls for both vertical and horizontal movements of the jaw and causes wearing of the teeth. Nature, has countered this by providing the horse with very long embedded teeth throughout the jaw and face. A relatively small part of the tooth is above the gum line at any time. The teeth erupt gradually throughout the horse's life to keep pace with the wearing down so that the surface of the teeth remain level.- Usually, that is. On occasion a molar, fails to oppose it's grinding mate, either from breaking or by delayed growth. This of course allows the opposing tooth to grow beyond the level of it's neighbors since it has failed to be worn down at the same rate. The resulting long tooth becomes more awkward and painful as it progresses. Eventually the owner notices that his horse is losing weight and dropping hay out of it's mouth in a wet ball instead of chewing and swallowing it. This is what brings it to the attention of a veterinarian.

Upon examination we often find a molar up to an 1½ inches longer than it's neighbors. The correction is straight forward and rather dramatic. We cut it off! A long tool that looks like a large wire cutter with compound action is used. Sensory nerves do not reach into the exposed tooth, so the action is painless though unpleasant. A mouth speculum is used to make the area accessible: Visibility is limited, The patient is definitely not like one of our species, mouth wide open on command, tongue voluntarily held out of the way and a bright light illuminating all parts. Instead we are looking into a long dark cavity with a big tongue often very much in the way. There is some resentment but fortunately we have sedatives that help both horse and operator. The stubby blades are worked around the offending tooth. The long handles are closed, sometimes with the help of a second party. A loud cracking noise is followed by the extra part of the tooth falling out of the mouth. A rasp like instrument is then used to smooth off any sharp points. Once or twice a year thereafter the offending tooth is rasped down to level before it becomes a repeat performance.

This problem was always met with a certain amount of satisfaction by me because the patient was in real trouble, the diagnosis was simple, the treatment was straight foreword, the relief was immediate and it was done with one visit. An ideal scenario for any veterinarian. One guy was so happy to have the long tooth out of his horse's mouth that he made it into a pendant to wear around his neck.

As a horse's teeth grow and wear down, enamel points are frequently left on the outside of the upper and inside of the lower arcades. This causes discomfort to the tongue and cheeks when chewing and can result in impaired food intake. The correction of this is called 'floating.' Simply put, it is grinding down the sharp points with a long handled rasp. I don't know why it is called floating but suspect that it is compared to the final 'floating' or smoothing out of fresh cement. There is no pain with the procedure, but some horses resent it. I imagine the grinding noise bouncing back and forth in their skull is hard to take.

I am sometimes asked how wild horses deal with these enamel points. I have no scientific answer, but I have two theories: One - they don't live as long as domesticated ones; and two - having no hay or grain available to them they must graze to eat. This may provide enough abrasive action to prevent the problem. Certainly no wild Mustang ever called to have his teeth floated. Which again points out the fact that Veterinary Medicine is never a one on one basis. There is always the third party.

MOST FAVORITE ANIMALS

My most favorite horse joined our family in a most unusual way. My assistant daughter and I were on a routine call to geld a horse. We had to wait awhile at the farm for the arrival of the owner, so we wandered over to a pasture fence to say "Hello" to a pretty headed friendly mare. Turns out she was a four year old Standard Bred, barely halter broke. The owner had been unable to train-her because of his advanced age. When the owner finally appeared at the fence, I remarked to him that she was a very pretty sociable sort of a mare. He said, "She's for sale." I said, "Let's get started with our work." I should have headed for my truck. He said, "You can have her for $100 and today's bill." At that moment a mosquito bit the back of my neck and perhaps I nodded my head to swat it. He claims I did. Anyhow acquiring another horse was the absolute farthest thing from my mind. My mind that day was on getting through our calls and getting home before dark. The subject was dropped. We did the surgery and headed out for other calls.

When we pulled into our farm in the late afternoon we were surprised to this same pretty head looking out of a stall whinnying for something to eat. Not wanting to lose a chance to place the mare, the owner had waited 'til we were out of sight, loaded her into his trailer, dumped her into one of our empty stalls, then disappeared before we reappeared. Before I had a chance to return her she worked her way into our affections and took up residence with us. My youngest daughter helped me train her to saddle. She threw us both several times before she settled into her new life style. I named her 'Temptation' after a polo pony I had leased while in college. She became a favorite trail horse and polo pony for many years. When she died twenty years later we were all saddened but thankful for the unusual way her previous owner had of horse dealing.

My most favorite dog was obtained in an equally unusual way. My sister-in-law bred Doberman Pinschers. Realizing that I was currently out of a dog, she asked me if I wanted a young Doberman. I said, "No thank you." The next day she opened the side door of my hospital and shoved this dog in, yelling, "If you don't want him after a week, I'll take him back." She was no fool. A week later, like the horse, we became bonded. For twelve years he became my best companion until his heart went into atrial fibrillation from over exertion on a trail ride. He learned to close doors, he learned to pick up litter on the floor and drop it in a waste basket on command. He accompanied me on farm calls. I forgot him once. As I pulled out of the drive, the owner of the farm yelled, "What do you want me to feed him?" He won a ribbon at a horse show for good behavior. His ashes are spread under a favorite tree of mine.

I often wonder what strange and benevolent force led these people to send me these initially unwanted very best animals.

Many times a client has presented a most favorite pet for treatment that wasn't obtained by design. It just wandered into their yard needing a home and a career of pethood.

THE REAL NEWS

Country Vets express their leisure time in many ways. This one has found there's no better way to waste time than messing around a sail boat. It was on my 22 foot sloop when the following happened.

Having slept the night on the my sloop, 'No Wake', with my Boxer dog, 'Teak', who incidentally enjoys his personal sleeping bag in the V birth, and having awakened before dawn, we hauled anchor and motored at trolling speed down the middle of the mirrored lake, as we were wont to do. Our destination was a port of call with a country store where we would add a newspaper and a cup of coffee to the ship's manifest. The sun was not yet up, but was clearly predicted by a golden rim decorating the mountain top. A mist hovered over the lake. Teak enjoyed the smells, being of the canine persuasion, while I, being of the human persuasion enjoyed the views. We both agreed that the moment was beautiful.

Suddenly over a mountain top there was a dramatic burst of sun rise. But as No Wake cleared the mountain the sun became completely eclipsed by a higher mountain. Before long however, the sun rose again with equal brilliance from behind the higher mountain.

We docked at the store, chatted with some local sailors about the weather and other nautical matters and soon commenced our return voyage.

There was now a favoring wind rippling the lake so we raised the jib and sailed as slowly as possible toward the home port. I read the paper while occasionally trimming the sail and correcting No Wake's course. The news was mixed, both good and not so good, but it occurred to me the real news that morning had been entirely missed. The real news for me was that given certain conditions with space, time, mountains and God, a dawn can actually have <u>two</u> sun rises.

Back the next day delivering health care to cows, horses and dogs, I felt quite satisfied with the 'real news' of the day before.

COWS ARE STUPID

Cows are stupid, loveable but stupid. Perhaps it's a good thing considering their life style. Why do I call them stupid? Because they eat nails. Horses are smarter. They have very sensitive lips. They feel and smell the food before swallowing. Foreign objects never pass these Equine sentinels. On the other hand our loveable cows just rake in the food with their tongue. Any unsavory object such as a nail or wire goes down unopposed and causes many cases of inflammatory indigestion, commonly called 'Hardware Disease'.

Cows are called Ruminants because the first of their four stomachs is called the Rumen. Sheep, Goats, Deer, Impala, Buffalo, Camels and many other species are also Ruminants. After the Rumen comes the Reticulum (commonly called Tripe and is often eaten), then comes the Omasum (commonly called the Butcher's Bible because it has several internal leaf like structures), finally the Abomasum which is the only true stomach and functions somewhat like ours with digestive enzymes. The Rumen churns the food then sends a bolus back to the mouth to be chewed again, commonly called 'chewing the cud'. The purpose of the first three stomach is to grind coarse feeds into a mash like mix where fermentation by friendly bacteria and protozoa can reduce the indigestible cellulose of grasses down to a digestible form of sugars. A truly magnificent example of symbiosis in which unlike organisms live together to their mutual advantage. This allows Ruminants to fill a big niche in the food chain. Meat eating Carnivors (wolves, coyotes, lions, etc.) and meat-plant eating Omnivors (humans) depend on ruminants and other herbivors to convert plant life to meat.

The farmer complains that his cow is 'off feed', her milk production is down and her manure is scanty. The examination reveals a low grade temperature. Her nose is dry instead of having the little beads of moisture of a healthy cow's nose. There may be signs of vomition in the manger. With a stethoscope we listen to her rumen noises. Normally the rumen makes beautiful noises like distant thunder. These may be absent. We suspect that she has a wire or nail lodged in her reticulum. The reticulum is located beneath the rumen and accepts heavier objects like little stones or nails, etc.. Next we rather rudely thrust a knee into her lower left abdomen looking for a grunt or other sign of pain. A White Blood Cell Count indicates the degree of infection and helps with the diagnosis. Putting all the symptoms together we make a probable diagnosis of 'hardware disease' and give the farmer three options. One - to sacrifice the cow; two - to operate; and three - to treat with a magnet. The third option will be described later. If he chooses to operate, then the fun begins.

We shave and scrub the left flank of the standing cow and inject scads of local anesthesia into the area. We then make an incision through the skin muscle and peritoneum into the abdomen. The peritoneum is a tough membrane lining the abdominal cavity.

The rumen is immediately encountered, opened and the edges temporarily attached to the skin to prevent escape of ingesta into the abdominal cavity. With a sleeve that extends to the shoulder we reach through the rumen down into the second stomach (reticulum). It is warm and gooey and mushy as we grope hopefully for the offending metal. Success means retracting a wire or nail and triumphantly showing it to the owner. If nothing is found it is a slow sad process putting the cow back together with the problem unresolved. There is no triumph in failure under the close scrutiny of the owner. This is when a veterinarian might wish he was a mechanic so he could just put in another part.

In the forties there was developed a technique for minimizing the damage done by swallowed nails. It involved the extraordinary procedure of installing a magnet into the second stomach using a 'balling gun'. A balling gun is a simple tool that accepts a big pill at one end with a ring at the other end that when plunged deposits a pill down the esophagus. The magnet being heavy, by passes the rumen to enter the reticulum. There it attracts ferrous metals to itself, preventing them from lodging in one place where they can cause irritation and possibly penetration of the stomach. It works wonders on all ferrous material, copper wire excluded. I used magnets on many cases of 'Hardware Disease'. I kept separate records and the recovery rate was fantastic. The number of surgery cases diminished.

The most important use of magnets however, is as a preventative tool. Instilled in a heifer, the magnets prevent most cases of the disease. As time went on it became important to avoid putting a second magnet into an animal. Two magnets decrease the magnetic force rather than increase it. How do we detect the presence of a magnet already in place? Easy! We run a compass back and forth under the cow's belly. If the needle goes crazy, there's a magnet already there. There was an occupational hazard connected with all this for me. My pocket watch kept stopping and my jeweler was getting tired of de-magnetizing it. This stopped when I kept the watch in another pocket. We put so many magnets into cows that it's a wonder they didn't all stick together and stop like my watch.

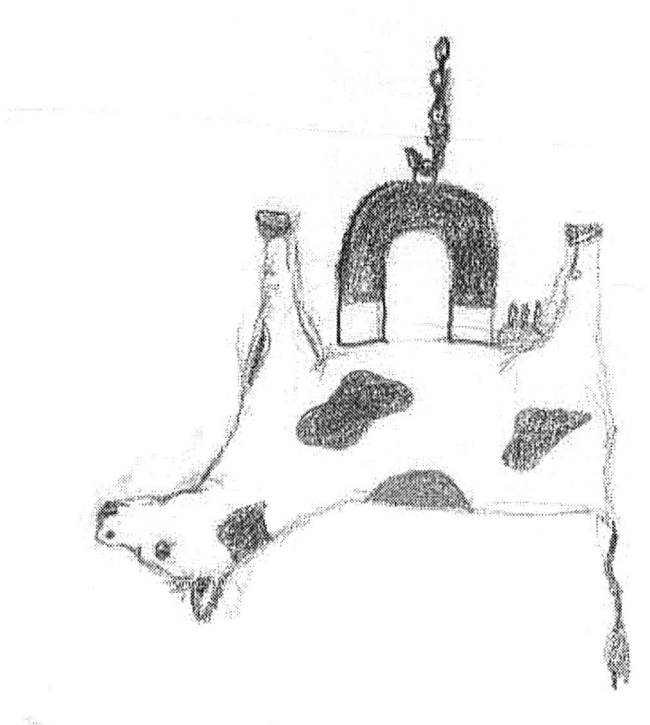

PURCHASE EXAMS

A second hand horse like a second hand car is generally examined before being purchased. It is called a 'Vet Check' or 'Purchase Exam'. The purchase exam for the vet is a real challenge and fraught with danger. We carefully go through the horse's systems of respiration, circulation, locomotion, teeth and sight. In some cases X-Rays, blood test and ultra sound are called for. Technically we are only concerned with health and soundness, but often we go further and evaluate the suitability of the horse for it's intended owner. Some observations are obvious and some are judgements. Some conditions of good health today can change in the near future. Occasionally if the health of the horse deteriorates weeks later the vet checker is suspect. Can you begin to see the dangers inherent in this business? To minimize these dangers we avoid the words 'pass' or 'reject'. It being wiser to point out the weak or strong points then give an evaluation of the capabilities of the horse considering the observed conditions. The decision can then be left to the prospective buyer. Sellers have been known to modify their horses' behavior with tranquilizers if they are too lively or with pain killers if they are hurting. Blood tests to rule out this possibility can be done. Over time I became rather proficient with these exams. I was able to satisfy my clients and protect my image with the seller when the sale was refused. My success with 'Purchase Exams' came to an abrupt end one regrettable day. It went like this.-

Rick was a horse dealer who had used my services for many years. We had seen him at horse shows and had played polo with him. I thought I knew him. I had 'Vet Checked' many prospective sales for him at his stable. This day was different. "Doc, I'm trucking a horse up state today. Can I stop at your Hospital for the exam and go on my way?" I realized it would be difficult to examine the horse in action in my parking lot but foolishly agreed. It is important to exercise a horse during an exam to check the heart and respiration and check for lameness.

Rick and horse arrived on schedule. I made a cursory exam of a nice little mare, had Rick jog her up and down my driveway for the heart and lung check, signed the form stating my opinions, and sent them on their way, feeling confident that the horse would be fine. After all Rick had said that she was ridden all winter without any trouble. Three days later the new owner called. She was upset. She said the mare was terribly asthmatic and had great difficulty breathing and that I should have observed this. I expressed my surprise and sympathy. I explained that if this be so, and I emphasized the 'if', it is the nature of asthma to be undetectable while in remission. It occurs only after contacting whatever agent they are allergic to. I advised that if she was dissatisfied she should return the mare and get her money back. I thought that would put closure on the disappointing affair. Not so!

She called me back the next day and for many days thereafter with increasing ire each time. It seems Rick was stalling on returning the money, claiming he had the horse on consignment and had already paid the owner, leaving him short. He could return only a fraction of the money. The unhappy owner continued her accusing calls and finally insisted that I should make up the difference of what Rick could not pay. That particular solution failed to gel with me. She then countered with a threat that she would report the incident to the Veterinary Grievance Board if I didn't comply. In order to stop the harassing phone calls I told her to do what ever brought her contentment.- Mistake!

Contentment for her meant carrying out her threat. I got the dreaded invitation to appear before the Grievance Board. The Board is made up of dedicated men who are willing to give up their time in an effort to maintain and improve the image and integrity of the Profession. They were interested in why I hadn't exercised the horse for the heart and respiratory exam. My feeble excuse was that a parking lot was a poor place for such an activity. However, I did point out that I had made Rick run the horse up and down my steep driveway several times. Rick was puffing pretty bad, but the horse did fine. This caused a chuckle and relieved the tension. Then the subject of the asthma that I could have missed was approached. I pointed out that Rick is a horse dealer, and as such his effort to put food on the table may call for fudging the facts from time to time, but he was most certainly not a fool. He would not be likely to sell a horse that he knew would come back with the return mail. A dissatisfied customer is time consuming and bad for a horse dealer's reputation. The Board properly reprimanded me for taking the path of least resistance and I accepted the criticism. Then came the zinger, they asked for records to prove that I had not received benefit from the seller in return for expediting the sale. I had no records for that-so they were left with a degree of suspicion. All I could do was to deny it and say that my code of ethics preceded our Grievance Board's existence and I wouldn't sell my soul for a few measly bucks.

A few months later I saw the mare for vaccinating purposes and she appeared normal.

Looking back on the affair, I see two possible scenarios. One – that the mare in her new environment experienced a combination of stress and allergens that indeed triggered an asthmatic attack. Or Two - That the new owner was unhappy with the horse and decided on a creative way to return it and get her money back. Both of which she eventually did, I hope to her complete contentment.

KETOSIS – REDUCING DIET

Under the stress of suddenly going into lactation, cows may develop a metabolic disorder labeled Ketosis. It is typified by a decreased appetite, scanty bowels, depression, decreased milk production and a very strange heavy breath odor resembling acetone. My assistant daughter complained that the heavy odor stuck in her nose for days. The name comes from the ketone bodies found in the blood and milk. It is essentially caused by the following chain of events. The metabolism of carbohydrates is interrupted by causes not completely understood. Carbohydrates are the precursor to glucose which is the body's primary source for energy. Being thus deprived of this source, the need for energy is compensated for ultimately by metabolism of the body fats. Rapid metabolism of the body fat results in an excess of a waste product of ketone bodies which are the cause of the symptoms and the name. The treatment is straight foreword and usually successful. An infusion of glucose, and or an injection of some form of cortisone is usually sufficient. The test for the disorder is easily done with the milk.

I was called to treat a cow that passed all the criteria for Ketosis. As I was giving the intravenous injection of glucosee I noticed that the automatic drinking bowl was dry and malfunctioning. The diagnosis was changed from Ketosis to dehydration and the treatment was changed to water which rapidly dispelled all the other symptoms. This was a clear but unusual cause for the interruption of carbohydrate metabolism.

Currently there is a popular reducing diet that calls for restriction of carbohydrate intake in order to call up metabolism of body fat. It appears that what is a disorder in cows has become useful for over weight humans, with a caveat against overdoing it to the point of producing ketosis. For those who find this diet useful let's remember that our bovine neighbors discovered it first.

OOPS OR AH HA S

In my practice I have often remarked in a more or less jocular vein - "We don't allow any 'Oops' here, only 'Ah Has'!"

Irreparable damage can be done by 'Oops' veterinarians. Constant vigilance is an absolute and can be long regretted if forgotten. Forgive me for plagiarizing, 'a mistake made in haste can be regretted at leisure.'

This happened to me. We had the sad order to put down two old horses. The request was firm. Arriving at the farm, the owner was not to be seen. Thinking she did not want to witness the procedure, we started. I always give a deep tranquilizer to minimize fear and anxiety. This was given to the first horse. I started to give the euthanasia solution when the owner appeared just in time to say that she had changed her mind.

This did not happen to me. It took place in a hospital where I was interning. -Two Wire Hair Terriers were entered on the same day. One was to be groomed and the other was to be euthanized because of a biting habit. He was mean. The kennel man inadvertently switched the two dogs in their kennels. You guessed it - the mean dog was groomed and the one to be groomed was put down. The veterinarian had the onerous task of discharging the dog, unaware of the mixup. He handed the mean dog to the owner of the one to be groomed. Whereupon the owner was bitten. The vet settled out of court.

This one happened, not to me, thank goodness. - The order was to castrate a bull calf. The vet arrived early. Not wanting to waste time, he assumed a bull calf tied in back of the cows was the subject and did the job. On his way out the owner appeared and said enthusiastically, "Before you go Doc, come in and see the bull calf I just bought to raise for a herd sire." You figure out the rest of the story.

LOOSE HORSE TRAGEDY

"What, oh that's terrible!" Carol had answered the last phone call of the evening. "Let me give you the doctor." The doctor frowned, not looking forward to an emergency at this time of night. It was a frantic call for help. Two horses had gotten out of their stall, gone on to a dirt road and been hit by a car. It was dark. It was cold. It was snowing. We went.

Most cases that I talk about are the successful ones. These are the easily remembered ones and may give the illusion that a country practice is all sweetness and light. The following experience should change all that.

As we hurried over the dirt road, I wondered if there was a better way to make a living, and I wondered at the resolve of my assistant to venture forth on such a call on such a night. Over a rise and around a curve we came on to the horror scene. Standing unsteadily in the middle of the road lit up by car lights was the first horse. A hundred feet into the woods lit up by flashlights was the second. We were urged to see him first and the reason soon became obvious. The victim's left front leg was broken and the skin and muscles were stripped away from the entire length of the upper leg bone. The horse was frightened and in great pain. He was in a completely hopeless situation for any chance of transporting or healing. We put him down on the spot on the cold dark snowy night. I believe he was buried where he fell.

We led the other horse about a mile to his home. Led is an exaggeration. He had to be pushed, pulled and supported all the way. It was a slow dreadful effort. He was bleeding internally. The barn had no lights, so to give intravenous fluids we had to work near the house. The fluids were warmed in the house but continued to freeze in the line. We took turns warming ourselves and the fluids in the house. Our efforts on this night were for naught. The horse died the next day.

It is always difficult to make a fair charge to the owner when there is a great loss like this. If we charge according to the time, expense and emergency status it would be unrealistic and we would often not be paid. I am usually satisfied if the expenses are covered. It is a lose-lose situation financially and emotionally that is best accepted as fact, then move on to the next case.

IKE THE RUNAWAY HORSE

Ike's reputation was not too good. He was a Thoroughbred Hunter who was easily spooked and had an aversion to jumping. He also resented being washed down after a work out. On this day while getting his bath after a workout he plotted to shorten the event. He was outside on a cross tie that was arranged between two adjacent barns. His plan went like this, "I'll pretend to spook at something, break loose and have some fun for a change." He did and his plan worked. One rope broke, the other pulled a board from the side of the barn. Ike left the scene as he had planned, but when he saw the board following him his instincts overpowered his judgement and told him it was a predator. He took off at a speed that no one realized he had. His plan had obviously gone wrong. He easily cleared a five foot fence and headed south down the road with the predator close behind. It was a Sunday summer afternoon and folks were generally relaxing on their front lawns. Seeing Ike galloping toward them at full speed with a plank dragging behind him roused their interest. So they stood on the edge of their lawns somewhat like one might view a parade, and watched. Ike disappeared down the road at a full gallop, unable to gain on his enemy. Next the watchers saw the owner and a couple barn help come running round the bend in hot pursuit. The good neighbors wanting to help, pointed with conviction in the direction the horse and plank had gone. This spurred on the chasers encouraged that they were not wasting their breath. Eventually Ike figured out what was going on. He had run farther than the Mountain Lion could anyhow, so he stopped to take advantage of some lush grass on a guy's lawn. That's where the breathless chasers picked him up with no trouble, and started back. The good neighbors now seeing a chance for some fun, applauded as Ike and the chasers minus the plank passed them on the return trip. The chasers took this in good spirit. In fact one of the barn help was seen to take a bow of acknowledgment to the applause.

After all was calmed down and the chasers realized that no people, cars or horses had been hurt, they began to see humor in the event. Firstly Ike had cleared a five foot fence dragging an anchor and revealed the fact that he really could jump, and secondly the folks excitedly directing traffic had helped change panic into good humor.

On a serious note, cross ties should be either strong enough to withstand the strongest pull or weak enough to break with a light pull. This is to prevent injury to a horse from tumbling over backwards if the ties break while he is pulling back.

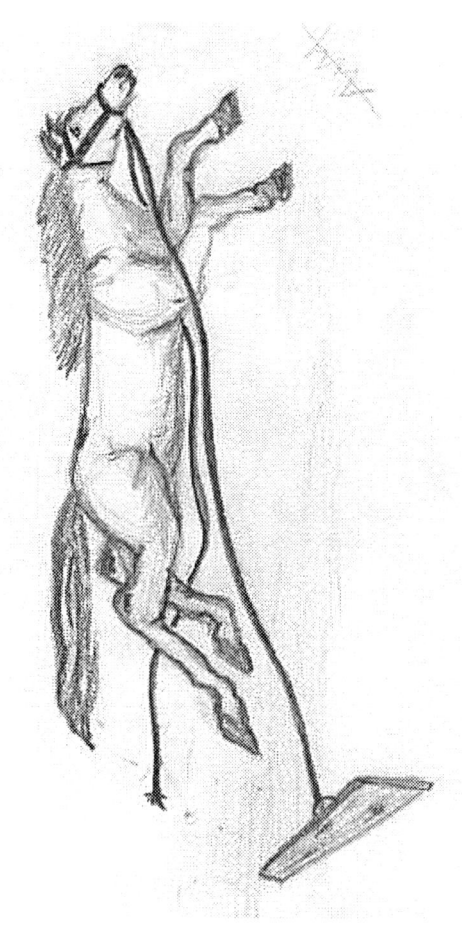

OH BOY IT'S STUCK

Emergencies are never pleasant, but some are less unpleasant than others.

For instance - " My dog is pawing at his mouth and he can't close it. He's drooling and he can't eat." We suspect what the trouble is and tell them to hurry him right down. When .the dog is on the table, we open his mouth and there it is - a stick across the top of his mouth wedged in between his upper molars. The trick of course is to remove the object, preferably without joining it. For this a tooth extracting forceps works very well. Usually without sedation, We make a quick move with the forceps and if the aim is good out comes the offending object. On the next page is a note from a little girl who really appreciated our good works.

The above scenario represents the outcome of most of these cases. However I recall one that wasn't quite so pleasant.

These owners were not very observant. Apparently the dog had the object stuck in place for a long time. The first thing they noticed was a foul odor from his mouth, which was the complaint that brought him to us. The wedged bone had put pressure on the roof of his mouth so long that it had created a hole into the nasal cavity. This turned out to be irreparable. For the rest of his life liquids emitted from his nose after drinking.

Dear Dr. Mills   Tues. 23

I will never forget when you took the bone from my dog chem's mouth. It was so nice of you.

We couldn't get it out. You must be magic. You are so kind.

Thanks a lot

Sincerely
Cheryl and Audrey Hanson

COMPASSION

The commendable virtue of human of compassion can sometimes go from humorous to unusual to extraordinary.

Humorous - My wife can catch flies in her hand. Does she crush them? No. She releases them outside.

Unusual - my receptionist said, "We have a walk in, claims he has an emergency." "Bring him in," I said. In came the biggest man you can imagine, at least 350 pounds. I couldn't see his patient at first because it was in the palm of his hand. While driving to work he had seen something moving beside the road. He stopped to investigate and found a starving, flea ridden kitten. Instead of tossing it aside, as others may have done, he hurried to the nearest vet to try to help it. I couldn't help feeling there was something unusual about a small hapless kitten being saved by a big macho man. Compassion runs in all sizes.

Extraordinary - We were overwhelmed by a compassionate woman who took it upon herself to solve the local feral cat problem. How did she go about this? She trapped them in 'Have a Heart' traps! She was a very good trapper. She brought them to us to neuter, check for feline leukemia, give Rabies vaccines and sometimes if they were ailing to put to sleep. The healthy ones she either tried to find homes for or released them in the area where they were caught. We did our work at a charge commensurate with her altruism. On occasion she brought in three cats at once. As soon as she freed up the traps she'd catch some more. Since these were wild cats they were hard to handle. We became proficient with our task without becoming victims of the program. We were able to anesthetize them while still in the traps and they were returned to the traps before they recovered. We devised a way to feed and clean them without removing them. They were returned to the good lady still in her traps. Since they were generally caught behind a restaurant it seemed there was no limit to her supply. We eventually became concerned that this compassionate person was becoming obsessed with her altruism to the point of self harm. She spent a lot of time and money on what appeared to be a 'finger in the dike' situation. One of my techs eventually made the comment, "I'll bet there's a couple guys surprised to see a little incision on their cat's belly." She was implying that some of the cats may not be entirely homeless.

It is well knows that the unwanted dog and cat population is a tragic problem. Responsible owners are the obvious solution, but fall short on the total situation. Animal Control People help by placing some from the pounds and euthanizing untold numbers, but this is necessity, not compassion. It's folks like our cat trapping lady and many others involved with homeless animals that qualify for compassion of the extraordinary type.

HORSE LAUGH

Electric fencing is designed to keep cattle and horses within an area, making conventional fencing unnecessary. When grounded by an animal that touches it, a pulsating intense but not dangerous shock is the result. The first shock is usually enough to remind the animal to keep it's distance. Having been electrocuted several times in my life by the evil wire, my approach is very respectful.

Springtime meant a rush to vaccinate horses against the so called 'Sleeping Sickness', Tetanus and various other diseases. Sleeping sickness (Encephalomyelitis) is a fatal nerve damaging disease of horses and humans. It is spread by mosquitoes apparently from a reservoir in wild water fowl. It is contagious to humans from the same source, but not from horse to human or horse to horse. Tetanus is also a nerve damaging disease. It is caused by bacteria (Clostridium Tetani) entering through a puncture wound where it produces a toxin under anaerobic (airless) environment. Horses are particularly susceptible probably because of the frequency of nails in their environment. Often the entrance wound cannot be found. Springtime vaccinating was always a rather pleasant seasonal activity for us. We saw many horses and owners that we might not see at any other time during the year.

On this memorable spring day we had vaccinated a stable of horses. Departing from the area we had to deal with an electric fence. My daughter handed me a tray of syringes, needles and vials while she skinned under the fence. She warned me to get down low and be careful. I replied rather testily that I was capable of handling myself without her advice. It was a foolish remark.

A nose clamp is a two foot long aluminum instrument used to control an upset horse by squeezing his nose. It is harmless and distracts the horse's attention for a short time to allow the vet to do a minor procedure. I put the clamp in my rear pocket. I got under the fence as advertised. The clamp didn't. It sent a bolt of electricity to my butt end that projected me forward on my face. My tray of things flew in all directions. My disrespectful daughter laughed so much that the owner warned her she might be fired. He didn't realize that she was cheap labor and had job security. As I was gathering myself together I distinctly heard a horse laugh coming from the stable.

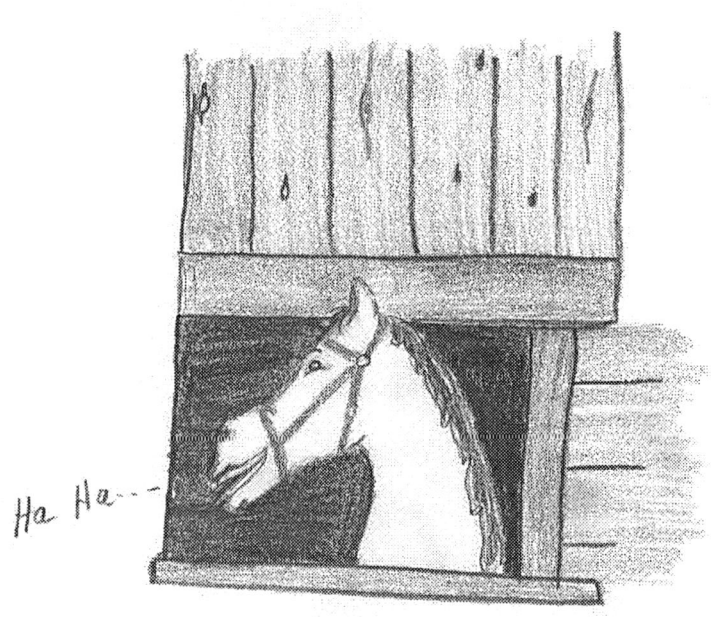

POPULATION EXPLOSION

Joanne paid us a visit. She was a cat lover among animal lovers in general. The conversation naturally turned to cats. This was her story, a true one.

Not long ago she was asked by a friend if she would take his cat that he was anxious to place in a good home. His landlord had mandated - no cats. "I don't want a cat now," Joanne said. "My old cat just died and I'm not ready." Time went by - then . "Joanne please reconsider, this is a super fine cat, how about it?" She weakened. "I'll think it over." Of course she eventually took the cat.

Time went by and Joanne became fond of the very fine cat. There developed however, an unchartered problem. The very fine cat was very definitely very pregnant. She added four female kittens to the household.

The gal who didn't want a cat now had five cats. They were cute and caused no particular problem at first. But shortly, as kittens are prone to do, they started to be cats. Joanne's husband began to pout and show resentment while Joanne showed a stiff upper lip and resisted. A compromise was sorely needed and fortunately reached. She could keep two kittens but none of the cats were to be let out of the house. Two were given away and two very fine kittens from a very fine queen cat were kept. There were now three cats in a household that hardly didn't even want one. However things settled down and peace in the family resumed. - One night somewhat later, the family was rudely awakened by weird sleep destroying howls coming from the cellar where the three female cats were kept at night. All the family members ran down to the scene armed with brooms and mops. The intruder turned out to be a tom cat who had found a hole in a cellar window. By some mischievous act of nature all three cats, mother and daughters were in heat at the same time (probably responding the to Wellesly Syndrome.) That was enough to attract males from miles around. The visiting tom was evicted with the mops and brooms scarcely missing his retreating tail, while the females were beaten back into their benevolent custody. Time went by and certain interesting things became obvious. Joanne, who was given to colorful language, put it bluntly, "He nailed all three of them!" Each very fine cat produced four very fine kittens. Now the gal who didn't want one cat had fifteen cats. Her husband's pouting progressed dangerously. Joanne took action to restore domestic tranquility. She placed the last twelve very fine kittens through great effort and pleading. Her friend, the source of all the population explosion was no help at all. None were put to sleep.

The moral of the story is obvious. Neutering of cats should be widely done. Joanne told her story for our amusement and indeed we laughed a lot. But we all know how serious the feral cat situation is. The answer is elusive and complex. It involves responsible owners, Animal Control People, and neutering both sexes. Spaying is an abdominal opening that requires time and concentration. Castration on the other hand is much less intensive. Of all the solutions to the feral cat problem castration should be the one that is pushed, mandated or subsidized to bring about greater acceptance.

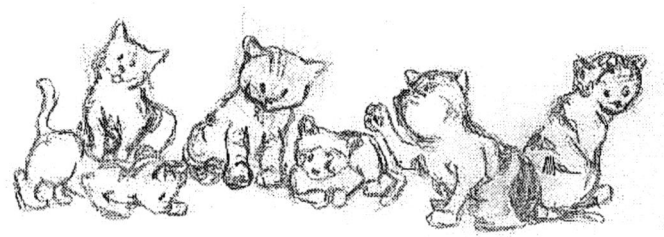

YOU KILLED MY CAT

"Good Morning - want coffee?" "Yes, thanks." The breakfast at the diner started off great. The regulars were there and our sometimes banter and sometimes serious talk was well underway. Things were slow so the waitress was apparently eager to start her own conversation.- "What kind of a doctor are you?" she asked. With some reluctance I admitted I was a veterinarian, thinking maybe I should be an undertaker or something that would terminate the conversation. "Oh," she said, "Are you the one on Worcester Street?" "Yes," I said hoping she'd mention some miracle cure I'd done. - No way. - "Then you must be the one who killed my cat." So much for the happy breakfast. She went on, "In the '78 blizzard my parents took my cat to you because he had been frost bitten in the storm, so you killed him."

That was 20 years ago. There must be a moral in this. Perhaps it illustrates the importance of a vet showing a considerate and compassionate approach to euthanasia. He may successfully treat a pet throughout it's life, but the final service of euthanasia is apt to be that which is remembered, especially by a child.

The breakfast was saved when the conversation turned to stories of the Blizzard of "78 which gave me a chance to restore my image.

DECISION TO EUTHANIZE

Veterinarians are frequently approached for advice as to when is the proper time to bring their pet's life to an end. This is a service we take very seriously. It is a privilege we have that human doctors do not have. When I am asked for this opinion, I am apt to suggest they deter the act when there is only loss of sight, hearing or teeth. In spite of these handicaps their pet can still communicate with the owner, they can enjoy being fed, or going for a short walk or ride. This can be a satisfactory relationship for both dog and owner. A dog's sense of smell is his strongest sense and persists after other senses fail. I'm sure you have all experienced your dog's cautious approach until his nose confirms what his eyes have seen. The joyous reunion waits for the scent recognition. The sense of smell and touch never fade. The feel and smell of a familiar hand can provide a path of communication with the owner long after the other senses have failed.

So at what point comes the sad decision? In my opinion it is when there is consistent pain, inability to rise from a resting position or incontinence of bowels and urine. These conditions reduce the quality of life for the dog and are so disturbing to the owner that the decision becomes logical and humane for all concerned.

I have been with many concerned owners preparing for the death of their pet. I count myself among them. Often they reach the decision only to back off. My advice usually is to stay on course. The agonizing decision will only have to be made again in the near future.

A client of mine handled this type of situation in a novel way. His failing old dog loved chicken, but was never allowed much at a time because it made him gassy. In fact after a bit too much chicken the old boy could easily clear a room. So this was the owner's plan. The night before the dog was to be put down he bought a roast chicken and allowed the dog to eat the entire thing with no restrictions. He passed away gassy but happy.

WHAT GOES ON HERE

She brought her cat in for a tune up. She was also anxious to unload some mixed feelings she had in regard to her cat. We listened - as we were prone to do, finding it sometimes more interesting than the subject at hand.. She said, "When my husband comes home, I'm lucky to get a low key 'Hi'. The cat on the other hand he showers with loving expressions like 'Tigger Dear, did you miss me? I'll get you your supper and you can sit on my lap while I read the paper." etc. etc. ad nauseum. Then she went on, "My husband has a bad back, it hurts him to bend over. The first thing he does,-there he is bending over the cat, rubbing its belly and apologizing for being late, sore back forgotten. I'm lucky to get a nod. What I want to know is, What goes on here?" She was actually in an up beat jocular mood through all this. She expected us to be amused and we were.

Times have changed. This morning the schedule called for a neutering. Not a bit unusual except that it was on a Pot Bellied Pig. Pigs as pets, can you imagine it? But perhaps it's not so strange. Pot Bellied Pigs are cute and have many appealing mannerisms. There may also be an unconscious appeal because physiologically pigs are not much different from humans from the head down that is. The internal organs are actually very similar to humans. Also we are both omnivorous (eat both meat and plant foods). I am reluctant to draw further parallels, but there are some.

Times have changed. In the fifties and sixties I was often engaged in castrating baby pigs and vaccinating them against Hog Cholera, hundreds of baby pigs. These were largely garbage fed pigs. The garbage had to be boiled for disease control. The garbage came from restaurants and homes. This made good use of all that food that we leave on our plates and is wasted. At these pigeries we would castrate dozens of baby pigs. Properly held, cut, vaccinate, release, back to eating. Pot Bellied pigs? -no way - appointment at hospital, anesthesia, sterile surgery, etc, etc. Times have changed.

ELECTRONIC BIRTHING

My daughter had a mare due to foal. She wanted to be there to give help if needed, but was regretting that it meant she had to get up in the night several times. She knew full well that in spite of her efforts the birth could happen in between her trips, making all her previous sleepless nights unnecessary.

Being thoroughly entrenched in the cutting edge of technology she came up with a device that when implanted across the mare's birth canal would give a signal when there was pressure applied to it, as in foaling. Being thoroughly entrenched in the old school and fond of the idea of the natural way of doing things, I was a reluctant implanter of the device. But my daughter is of the disposition that it is easier to go along with her than to resist.

These are the events of an electronic foaling - My daughter and her husband were out of town. The housekeeper was made aware of the possible event.

Mare starts foaling. Implant gives off it's signal.

Signal is picked up by intercom between barn and house.

Housekeeper hears signal. Calls my daughter on the cellular phone in her car.

Daughter calls trusted friend from her car. Friend gets out of bed and hurries to the scene.

Perhaps I should mention here that the mare was bred artificially. So far as I know there was no genetic engineering or in vitro fertilization. After the first cell division nature was allowed to take over unmodified by modern technology.

I am barely accepting the ways of the twentieth century and here we are in the twenty-first. Luxuries soon become necessities. I am probably the last one to admit it, but last isn't never.

19TH CENTURY PREFERRED

Monty was a Standard Bred whose occupation was pulling a One Horse Shay around Old Sturbridge Village, round and round all day every day all summer. Old Sturbridge Village is a living museum in Sturbridge, Mass. It relives life and times of the early 19th century. Monty loved his job and his owner was good at portraying an early 19th century gentleman. The visitors loved them and all was well,- until.

"Doc will you take this call, the Village is calling about a sick horse, they seem quite anxious?" I answered the phone and the owner-driver explained that Monty had a bad eye and was shying away from people on that side, making him a bit dangerous to use in public. My wife occasionally went with me on calls and she was eager to go on this one. Cars were strictly forbidden in the Village, so we were told to meet the owner at the Welcome Building and plan to walk from there. Monty, his owner dressed in early 19th century clothes and the One Horse Shay met us as planned. I made a cursory exam of the eye and suggested that we repair to a dark barn for a better exam with the opthalmascope. Looking into a hores's eye in the sunlight usually gives the observer a distorted reflection of himself rather than a look into the patient's eye. The logistics of getting to the dark barn is perhaps the gist of this story. A One Horse Shay is designed for one horse and two people. Guess who walked. I found myself slugging along in the dust carrying some of my equipment while trying to keep up to Monty and his two passengers. My wife would look back from time to time with an odd smile to check up on me, then return to enjoying the scenery of the outdoor museum. Monty's eye responded to treatment nicely and we saw quite a bit of each other afterwards when it came time for annual vaccinations, worming, teeth floating and such. But the doctor patient relationship was strained because Monty never really liked me. I think he would have preferred a 19th century doctor who wouldn't stick a needle into his upper eye lid.

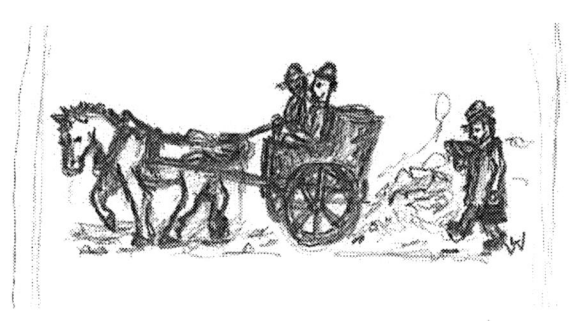

BREECH

It is very gratifying to take part in the miracle of birth of a calf, especially one that needs help. On a cold day the calf will appear steaming like water on a hot rock, balling and eager for life.

It's 4:30 - in the morning, 10 degrees and snowing. Our dairy farmer rolls out of bed, grabs a coffee and struggles to the barn. He turns on the lights, the cows are up and calling for their feed. He stops at a pen where he has an expectant heifer.

It's 5:30 AM - and my phone rings. "I've got one having trouble calving Doc. Can you make it?"

I was always eager to get a dystocia (difficult calving) call. It pleased me because the problem was clear cut the animal was in great distress, the diagnosis was simple, and the solution was mechanical. Successful or not, the problem was finalized with one visit and there was no burdensome decision to identify the disease and formulate a treatment. After a delivery our first effort is to clear the throat of mucous, then place the calf in front of the mother, who eagerly cleans it with her tongue. This invigorates the calf and starts the bonding. With dairy cows, however, the bonding is short lived. The calf is allowed the colostrum (first milk) then separated and hand fed to allow the dam's milk to be sold. The colostrum is important to the calf because of its increased content of vitamins, minerals and immune factors.

It's 6:30 AM - and I get there about the same time my heater starts putting out warmth. The cow is down and obviously exhausted. She has been trying to calve for hours. We help her up, I tie the tail out of the way, wash her rear, put on a shoulder length sleeve and make the examination. It's a breech.

In a normal presentation the front feet appear first with the head resting between the legs. If one or both of the legs or the head is turned back the parturition cannot proceed until these are returned to a normal position. In a posterior presentation the rear feet appear first. Calving is possible in this position but more dangerous because the breathing end is the last to appear. A posterior presentation with the legs mal- positioned foreword is a breech. It is a difficult dystocia and cannot proceed until corrected. The examination on this morning is discouraging. The calf is large in relation to the pelvis and the lubricating uterine fluids are scant due to her long effort at calving. Attempts to correct the mal-position are futile. It's time to give the farmer some options.

One - to attempt a delivery which may not be successful and would mean a dead calf and possibly an injured cow. Two - to sell the heifer and minimize the loss. Or - three to do a Caesarean section thereby increasing the chance of a live calf and cow. The farmer opts for the surgery and the fun begins.

Caesarean sections are done on the standing animal when possible. I shave and scrub the right flank and inject local anesthesia. An incision is made through the skin, muscle, fascia and peritoneum. The uterus is immediately available. I open the uterus on to the pulsating calf. The placenta is opened and an obstetrical chain is attached to a leg. Now I have the problem of a 50 to 100 pound calf that must be lifted up and out. Not being strong enough for that I attach ice tongs to a rafter and with a small block and tackle running from the ice tongs, I deliver the calf to its new environment. The calf is attended to by the farmer while I suture the uterus, muscles and skin. I inject a drug to help the uterus contract. The placenta is removed and I give intravenous fluids and antibiotics. By now the cow and calf are introduced. I chat with farmer about the weather and the price of milk while the calf takes it's first milk.

It's 11:AM - The day will be long but my feelings of accomplishment for the cow, calf, farmer and myself will make it a pleasant long day.

PREVENTIVE MEDICINE

In our practice we send reminder cards to encourage owners to keep up with their pets' preventive medicine. Preventive medicine is perhaps the most valuable phase of this business. The problem is however that one never knows what he got for his money. Medicine that affects a cure is obviously worth it. Medicine designed to prevent a sickness that may not happen is a harder sell.

Let me tell you about a patient that had no use for preventive medicine. He was sitting on his master's lap while they read the evening paper and the mail together. The junk mail was disposed of without event, then came a post card. What was that awful smell? - The pup was out of there in a flash and took refuge behind the refrigerator. It was one of our reminder cards, he recognized the smell and wanted no part of it. In spite of his pleading the pup ended up getting his non sick preventative medicine.

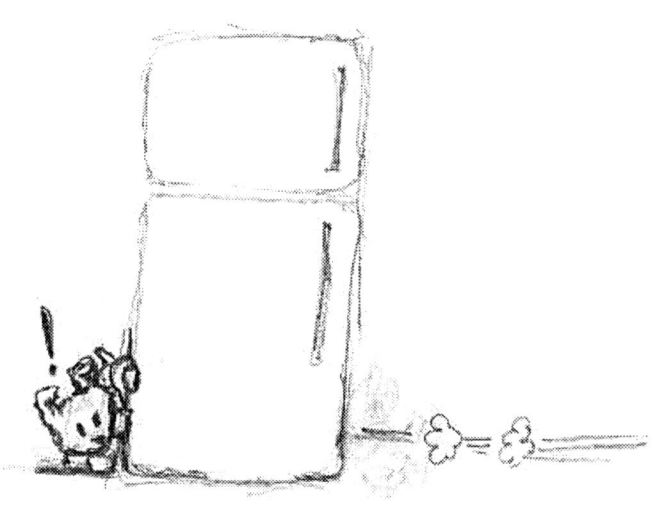

ALL IN A DAY'S WORK

She came into the office with an Iguana. A dish had fallen on one of his toes and it was dislocated. We reduced the dislocation and fashioned a splint for it. This gal was super fond of her reptile. She made a remark that amused my wife. She said, "You can't believe how much I love this Iguana, and to think I almost bought a dog."

- - - - - - - - - - -

The heavy draft horse continually stomped his rear feet, which was the reason I was called. I was pleased to discovered he was supporting a family of heel mites which were quite easily cured. In making the diagnosis, I was holding his rear foot up to get a skin scraping. The horse moved his leg in protest. The owner remarked, "Don't mind him Doc, if he kicks you I'll hit him with a shovel."

- - - - - - - - - - -

It was the time of year when we traditionally showed appreciation to the mail man for faithfully delivering many catalogues on a daily basis, catalogues that often pushed the dumpster over the top. It was Christmas so I put a nice big Chedder Cheese package into the mail box. Simple enough except that vibration of the road caused the cheese to fall out on to the shoulder, whereupon the mailman instead of receiving a present ran over it. The injured cheese was rushed into the hospital. The wound was debrided and cleaned. The healthy part of the cheese was being eaten by the frugal staff members when in came a more particular sort who, upon witnessing the scene screamed, "Ugh, you're eating road kill!"

PROUD OF HIS SCARS

He was an older happy spirited sort of a man, thoroughly extroverted and uninhibited. When he and his LLasa Apso bounced into my office my first impression was that they weren't really matched. I would have expected this type of guy to have a Dalmation or a Weimaraner. He started by recounting loudly for me and the whole waiting room to hear that I had neutered the dog and had to open up his whole belly to find the second testicle, then added that he had not changed his name after he was castrated.

The LLappsa Appso was on the exam table for his up-dating. As I was examining his teeth the man commented, "He bites his owner." "He does!" I said, "Who's his owner?" "I am, you should see my scars." He was actually proud of the scars on his arms which he expected me to admire. I heard a subdued chuckle from my tech as I cut short the teeth cleaning. I asked, "Is he a good companion for you, does he like to ride around in the car or go on walks with you?" "Oh yes, we're buddies most of the time, except when he bites me. You know when you're petting your dog it lowers your blood pressure." I agreed. " I've had three heart attacks, but I can handle them," he said. I asked if the Llassa Appsa helped him handle his heart attacks. "Oh yes," he said, "sometimes he lowers my blood pressure but sometimes he raises it. "It was obvious to me that omitting the biting episodes, they loved each other. They proudly paraded out of the office looking for new adventures.

- - - - - - - - - - -

Some office calls necessarily take longer than others. This is understood, but we try to avoid a back up in the office. Mrs. Wood had the courtesy to call and warn me that her office call would take more than average time. "That's OK," I said, "What's up?" "Well", she said, "I'm going to bring two horses, two cats and three dogs." Using her horse trailer, cat carriers and the back seat of her car she brought them all and it did take a bit longer than usual.

- - - - - - - - - - -

Speaking of horse trailers, sometimes they are used for dogs. Donna's dog was so big and arthritic that she couldn't get him up into her car. Undeterred, she pushed him up the ramp of her horse trailer and pulled into the parking lot quite as though it was the normal thing to do.

- - - - - - - - - - - - -

"Mrs. Martin, your dog is too fat." I must have said that a million times and then discussed ways to reduce the pet's weight. Very few ever took my advice, it's just too much fun to feed a dog. "What can I do?", she asked. "Well," I said, "you could start by feeding him once a day." "I do," she said, "I start in the morning and stop at night." Obviously she had no interest in having her dog look any different than she did. They were both fat and happy.

- - - - - - - - - - -

The poor dog had not responded to my efforts to relieve his constant all body itch. He had lost most of his hair. His skin was thick and scaly. His thumping elbow kept his folks awake at night. The owners, the dog and I were getting desperate for some relief. The itchy dog had his own bed, a horse hair couch.

The time came when the people sold their house. They left the horse hair couch behind. The dog recovered and we came to the conclusion, rather late, that he had had a contact allergy to his horse hair couch.

I was late in diagnosing the condition. But learned what advice to give the next time. Simple - sell your house.

- - - - - - - - - - - - - -

Alone at the hospital one evening I decided to answer the phone instead of letting the answering machine handle it. "This is Officer Jones at the police station, we have a dog here with your Rabies tag on it". He gave me the number and I was able to give him the dog's address and phone number. I was pleased to be able to help and dismissed the subject. The phone rang again. "It's me again, looks like this dog is going to keep me company all night, can you give me his name?" I gave him his name and told him what he liked for supper.

SADDLE BAG CALL

In the 50's we had bigger snow storms and smaller snow plows. The combination of which often resulted in blocked roads for days at a time a situation that had little influence on the timing of bovine illness.

Not wanting to be denied of my chance to deliver our motto of 'Cure for Some, Help for Many , Comfort for All' health care to the cows, I found an alternate way of transport. A friend and client had a little 15 hand gray horse called Silver Spray that he willingly loaned me. The saddle bags were loaded with everything that I thought would be needed for the occasion, realizing that any omission would be awkward indeed. Arriving on horse back was always met with appreciation by the worried owner and a hero like attitude by me.

- - - - - - - - - - -

I have a stray cat that I want to keep. Will you spay and vaccinate it for me at a discount?", she asked over the phone. "But if you want to keep the cat, it's no longer a stray," I said. "Oh," she said, "I'm having such a difficult time, I have to work two jobs just to make Bingo money." She called three times during the day, taking about ten minutes each time. During the course of the last call it was revealed that the stray cat status ended a year ago when she took it in. During that time it had had a litter of kittens. This amused us so much that we agreed to a discount just to reward her deceptive resourcefulness.

- - - - - - - - - - - - - - - -

As I pulled into the driveway on a horse call for a new client, the owner came out of his house and handed me a two dollar bill. "Thanks," I said, "But you don't have to pay in advance." "I owe it to you," he said. "How come?" "Well," he said, "16 years ago I was two dollars short on your bill for castrating my cat. You said to pay me the next time I saw you. This is it" You can bet that made my day. Incidentally, if it went back another 16 years, the 2 dollars could have taken care of the entire bill.

BITE-THE BULLET

"Good Morning, the Daniels Farm called this morning. They have a cow that's coughing and off feed." This had the potential for an emergency, so I hurried through the small animal cases. When I entered the barn I sensed trouble. There was more than one cow coughing. I ran a temperature check of the herd and found three quarters of them elevated. This was a situation that all vets and farmers dreaded, a herd endemic. The problem was complex. Treatment was labor intensive and expensive being an intravenous injections of every sick cow, every day. The cows dropped in production, deaths were possible, and the farmer's expenses increased while his income went down. The vet had no choice but to use large quantities of medicine and time with the prospect of a long wait for return on the cost of drugs and time. There was no choice but to bite the bullet, as we did when it became necessary.

FRED'S OLD WOODEN BARN

Fred was a big, rough cut, friendly dairyman, with hands as big as the side of a cow's head. He had taken over his father's farm when it became too much for the older man. This was the way it was in those days. Handing down the farm to the next generation. It is rare now. I was pleased when Fred took over the farm, his father was not quite as friendly. In fact he had thrown me off the farm at an earlier date. As the Town Milk Inspector I had shown up at his door to announce that I was there to inspect his dairy. The old man wanted no part of this young stranger invading his fiefdom. He ordered me off his property. We eventually developed a working relationship, and I would often go home with a dozen eggs after working on his cows. Still I was more comfortable working with Fred. His friendly good humor was contagious. He often invited us into the house to chat with his elderly mother before we left.

It was lucky for me my daughter was small and never timid around animals, nor were they timid around her. For instance often when I tried to lead a horse out of a stall I would go round and round reaching for the halter succeeding only in getting the horse's rear end in my face. My daughter, on the other hand, could have a horse out and on the crossties by the time I made my first go round.

She was the same with cows. In a big old wooden barn like Fred's that came in handy. These ancient barns had many interesting features. Behind the cows were scuttles which hinged so they could be lifted up to allow the farmer to hoe the manure down below. In the spring it was a laborious ritual to shovel out a winter's worth of manure to spread on the fields. At the cows' heads were the mangers. These were closed in by hinged boards to preserve body heat. They could be lifted up for feeding. There was very little room between the cows' heads and the boards in front of the mangers. This worked just fine for feeding the cows and keeping the barn warm. But it left the veterinarian to fend for himself. Any blood testing or other treatments that needed to be done around the head meant that someone had crawl into the manger between the many heads of cows to set the nose leads or do any other administrations. This person was then bumped by horns at one end and scraped by rough tongues at the other end. I regularly volunteered my daughter for this task. She sputters about it to this day.

Those older, open rafted all wooden barns have phased from the scene, replaced by covered walls and ceilings, automatic gutter cleaners and other conveniences. This of course is to enhance the production of cleaner milk. One old time client of mine with an old fashioned wooden barn had his milk room walls covered with 'Clean Milk Certificates'. This points out that the production of clean milk depends as much on the milker as on than the barn.

EXPECT THE UNEXPECTED

On an ordinary routine day the phone rang and gave me an ordinary routine order to geld a horse. Routine? Hardly! The horse was a Western Mustang, completely unbroken.

During this time the Government in an effort to control the population of wild Mustangs developed a system of selling individual animals to qualified people. The man calling for help this day was one of the qualified people.

This case presented a problem. The horse was in a corral obviously half wild. The owner was an Eastern cowboy type. He lassoed the horse on the second try and snubbed him to a post. Then it was my turn. The gate was on the other side so I had to climb over the corral fence. The Mustang was struggling at the end of the rope making it dangerous to approach. An intravenous injection was out of the question, so I waited until he paused to catch his breath and with an extra large dose of sedative I moved in to give him an injection in the rear. The increased sedative dose eventually worked, making an intravenous jugular vein catheter for anesthesia possible. My assistant daughter passed the instruments through the rails. After the surgery I took advantage of the situation to trim some very long hooves. They had over grown during confinement. He obviously wasn't a suitable subject for trimming by traditional ways. I climbed back through the rails and headed out feeling very Western while no doubt the horse was beginning to feel quite Eastern.

An immense truck filled the parking lot one morning. There is one prevailing characteristic in the life of a country vet - you never know what unusual event the day may bring. You only know that it will probably happen. Out of this large van came not one but twelve donkeys. They had developed an intolerable itch. They were scratching themselves with their feet and tongues, they were rubbing against each other, they were miserable. To make matters worse, they were scheduled to be ridden for a basketball game that night. Their business was to have students ride them in a gym with special soft shoes for a rollicking game of basketball. We suspected a form of mange, but the sudden onset of them all suffering from the symptoms at once and the failure to demonstrate any mites under the microscope weakened that theory. They were dirty so with our hose and gallons of therapeutic soap they were given a thorough bath. They dried in the sun and performed that night without incident.

The expected unexpected thing happened again recently. While relaxing in the evening one of the few clients that have our home phone number called with the urgent complaint that

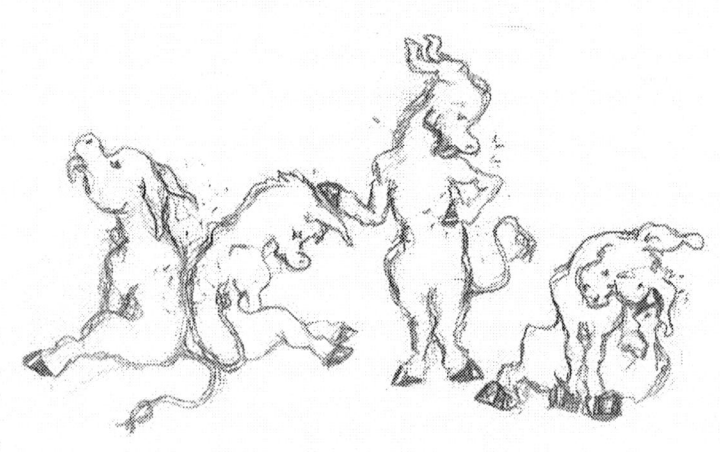

Itching Donkeys

one of her Sheltie dogs was in severe dystocia. She is a long time client who has bred quality Shelties for many years. I knew that she wouldn't make a foolish call for help, so I responded and she helped me with a Caesarian section which she has done in the past. The bitch had had one live vigorous pup, but the second one was grossly over sized and dead. Surgery was the only solution to her problem. This provided the unexpected event of the day.

THE SHOW MUST GO ON

In a hail storm the average person can run for cover or at least put on some rain gear. In the Veterinary Profession I discovered that it ain't necessarily so. Here's how I found out.

One apparently fine summer day we were engaged in gelding an Appaloosa colt in the field. We had the patient under anesthesia in preparation for the procedure. That's when the storm broke, a hail storm of unusual proportions. My wife ran for a blanket to put over the horse, not over me. I was committed to proceed with the operation which I did as quickly as possible. When I stood up afterwards I found my rear pockets full of ice. Such are the occasional vicissitudes of country Veterinary practice. Human surgeons take notice.

THESE ARE YOUR PUPS

"Hi, what can I do for you?" she said as she opened the door. "These are yours." said the visitor, and she put down a basket full of puppies. "What do you mean, I don't want any puppies. How come they're mine?"." "Well," the visitor said, "Your dog is the father, he came into our yard and bred our female. We didn't want her to have pups, so they're yours." Rather than put up a fight she took the little illegitimates, raised them, and found homes for all but one. The one she kept turned into a fine dog, in fact they all did, but that isn't the point of the story. What I would like to suggest is that the owner of a bitch in heat has a considerable responsibility to keep her out of reach of males eager to put their genes into the next generation. This is not easy considering the three week duration of most heat periods. Male dogs can detect the scent of estrus for miles around and readily leave the comfort of their homes to follow their instincts.

Don was the unofficial mayor of our neighborhood. He was regarded as mentally challenged and he was proud of it. He was challenging all right with his basic wisdom and wit. He couldn't read, but somehow got a driver's license. He drove his car at a crawl at all times, piling up impatient drivers behind him. Don couldn't write but he did have a trade mark, his feet. His feet were at right angles to his forward direction. It was easy to tell where he had been after a snow fall. Don loved his beer. One night he was stopped for erratic driving. Telling me about it, he said, "Doc, the cop stuck his flashlight into my one good eye and told me to get out and walk a straight line. Heck Doc, I can't walk a straight line when I'm sober." His license was lifted for a time but he solved the problem by driving his lawn mower down town at roughly the same speed he did his car. Don had a good memory in spite of the mental challenge. When on occasion he played cards with us he was really good. Once I complimented him on his memory. He said, "Oh yes, I have a memory like a - a - what do you call that animal with a long trunk?" He loved it when we laughed at him, but I doubt if he knew why we were laughing.

I was surprised one day to see Don waddling into our yard quite obviously in a truculent mood. "Doc," he growled, "We've been neighbors for a long time with no trouble, but Rud has got to stay out of our yard." Rud, my Doberman Pinscher, was generally a home body. "OK," I said, "I'll have a talk with him and see what the trouble is." It developed that Don's female Doberman was tied in the yard while in heat. Rud's pups were well on the way. Unaccountably Don became his old sweet self after his dog began to show her condition. A little research revealed that he was getting offers to buy the pups. Rud was a rather well known dog. In fact he was probably the only dog to win a prize at a horse show. He won it for good behavior. Folks wanted his pups. These pups became valuable family members for years to come.

I'm defeating my purpose with these stories of mismated pregnacies that turned out to be a success. I had intended to encourage people to house their dogs while in estrus, to keep peace in the neighborhoods.

SIT ON THE HEAD

"My horse has trouble chewing food and he's losing weight." This is a frequent complaint with middle age and older horses. Our thoughts ran through the possibilities of worms or bad teeth before considering more complicated things like infection or organ failure. In this case it quickly became obvious that it was his teeth. Upon examination we found that his lower jaw extended far beyond his upper jaw.

Horses teeth grow throughout their life. Normally the rate of growth is worn down evenly by the opposing teeth. When there is no opposing tooth it is easy to see the potential problem of a long tooth developing. This unfortunate animal had long molars and his lower incisors were out of control. Remember the lower jaw was projected foreword, so the lower incisors had no opposing grinders and were free to grow uninhibited, for the same reason the lower first molars were free to grow too long. Concurrently since the entire lower arcade was moved forward, the last upper molars found no opposing teeth and were also too long. If not corrected, the teeth eventually would impact the opposite gums with obvious painful results.

Experienced horseman know that if a horse is down and you want to keep him down you lay your body across his head. Horses always get up front end first. (Cows, on the other hand, get up rear end first.)

Sitting on the horse's head forces him to stay down, unless he is unusually strong, or the body across his head is unusually light.

This day we set out to even up some molars that resembled a mountain range. This would have been routine except for the unwanted assistance of the owner who was well indoctrinated with the 'sit on the head system.' The methods for doing this type of dental work are described in another episode labeled

'Long Tooth.' This case deals more with the owner than the horse's teeth. The project called for general anesthesia. We had the patient recumbent on the arena floor with nice access to his Jugular vein by means of an indwelling catheter. This was important for giving fluids or more anesthesia when needed. It promised to be a long job.

As I turned around for some equipment, the horse raised his head indicating the anesthesia was light and calling for more pentathol to be added to the fluids already flowing. The owner responding to the age old tradition, jumped on his head. His quick reaction was understandable, but in so doing his foot removed the catheter from the vein and buried it in the bottom of the arena. Now we had a 1.000 pound horse half anesthetized and in no mood to hold still for repositioning another catheter. The prospect of letting him recover only to put him under anesthesia again was unacceptable and there was no time for me to run for the books to look up 'half anesthetized horse'. To the rescue came my favorite short acting anesthesia. With trepidation I loaded a syringe and luckily was able to inject it into a vein that was a moving target. This restored control until we could start over again, somewhat shaken.

On the return trip my assistant, who had an active imagination questioned, "What would happen to a horse like that in the wild, without vets foolish enough to come to the rescue?" This gave me a chance to expound to my captive audience about how nature evolved the very functional horse. "In the first place," I replied, "a horse with that type of genetic failure would not survive, he would be counted among the small and weak and be suitable prey for Mountain Lions or Wolves. Mutations are slight changes in the genetic programming of an animal, some are beneficial and some are deleterious (harmful). This would have been an example of a harmful mutation, and by nature's way, be eliminated before reproduction age was attained. The harmful change would thereby be halted in it's tracks. In the case of a beneficial genetic change the fortunate recipient would prosper and therefore more readily add the change to the genetic pool. In time the advantageous change would become established in the species, whereas the deleterious one would disappear." My assistant by now was sound asleep dreaming no doubt about how a wild horse would go to a dentist.

BIG HEARTED SOULS - SMALL MINDED SOULS

In our society there are many big hearted souls who just can't resist rescuing stray or feral cats. They are however out numbered by many small minded souls who insist on dropping off unwanted cats or kittens to fend for themselves. If they live as feral cats they hunt, promote food from wherever they can and add to the problem by multiplying. In any case there is considerable suffering and disruption of the bird population. The bighearted souls are part of the solution, the small minded guys are part of the problem. Well intended folks occasionally get out of control and inadvertently create another problem. It is usually a lonely older person who starts by befriending a stray cat with food and shelter. The cat soon tells his indigent friends and before long there are many tenants keeping the human host company. I have seen such homes literally overrun with cats; cats on the tables, cats on the chairs, cats on the shelves and beds, cats, cats cats; with hygiene and odor completely out of control. It creates an unhealthy environment for cats and man. Cats are by nature solitary. In their wild natural state all cat species are loners except for the small Lion prides. Too many cats in a household are at serious risk for diseases such as Viral Leukemia, upper respiratory tract infections, parasites, etc. As veterinarians we often have to figuratively take these kind older folks by the hand and gently but firmly impress on them the necessity of not over doing it. Many of these unfortunate cats must be euthanized by vets or Animal Control People in order to make these souls be part of the solution.

At the risk of offending some folks who may think we are cruel, I'm inclined to tell a stray cat story. It involves a 'part of the solution' family who had a small farm. They loved animals, they were compulsive cat rescuers. They had well over 20 cats on their place. I chided them for letting them multiply. I agreed to neuter them at half price if they promised to euthanize any new recruits or place them elsewhere after being neutered. They agreed and the plan went well with many being neutered and regrettably an occasional cat being euthanasized. This tale is about a very wild female who had taken up residence in their barn. They brought her in to be spayed. We soon found out she was an escape artist. Her first escape came about because our kennel girl tried to befriend her. She opened the kennel door a crack in order to pat her, and zip, the cat was out. I say 'zip' because that's the only way to describe it, the action was too fast for the human eye to see. There are some old home made wooden kennels that we have kept because they are big and comfortable for large older dogs. She holed up under one of these big wooden kennels. The next morning the kennel girl said she had retrieved the cat from under the kennel with the noose, put it back in the kennel and before she could close the door, zip - out again. The next morning she told me the cat was hiding next to a wall behind the stretcher. "OK", I said, "We've got her this time. I'll take charge!" I took a fish net which is useful for entrapping a hysterical cat that is threatening to use up all our band aids. I said to her, "Enough of this nonsense, watch me handle her. Slowly move the stretcher and I'll catch it with the net." She did and I did - almost. The net pounced, completely covering the escapee, completely except for the nose. Zip - gone again. It reminded me of the saying, 'A camel's nose under the tent is soon followed by the rest of the camel.' Back under the big kennel. "What was I supposed to watch?" the girl said. Next day we got out the big guns. We sprayed the cat with a hose in order to flush her out. The girls were waiting at the other end with the net. I heard the victory cry, "We've got her." Back in the kennel. The cat was in a dangerous state of mind. I decided to go ahead with the spay. She was netted again in order to give the anesthetizing injection. In the split second that was necessary to remove the net, you guessed it, zip - out again, making fools out of all of us. Back under the big kennel, only this time she passed out from the anesthesia, out of reach. Panic! We finally retrieved her and she was spayed. She was kept in a sky kennel thereafter. When the owner came for her and he wanted to transfer her into his own sky kennel we said, "No thank you," and gladly gave him ours. The cat is now living a happy 'part of the solution' life.

In a serious vein, feral cats are a growing ecological problem. The solution has several avenues, responsible owners who prevent their cat from being bred is an obvious one. Spaying is an obvious help. The surgery however involves an abdominal opening and tends to be too expensive for some. Spay clinics are a help. Neutering males is less involved and less expensive and should be widely done.

HORSE SHOW VET

Being a horse show vet can be either harrowing or ego inflating but never boring, especially if you have three daughters competing at the same show. The ego part is probably due to the continual calling for you over the loud speaker system. The harrowing parts are many. For one or two, read on.

My daughters took to horse showing like ducks take to water. The logistics of this required a good alarm clock, plenty of gasoline and a budget adjustment that called for a trade off of many amenities for entrance fees, trailers and vans, etc.

In the 50's and 60's the sudden appearance of companion horses in every back yard caught the equine vets in short supply. Most vets in our area wouldn't go within ten feet of a horse. I wasn't that careful. When the horse show managers discovered there was a vet on the grounds, they nailed me, and I served as a show vet for many years. There were rules against show officials having family competing in the same show, but the managers fudged in my case because there were so few vets to choose from in our area. The harrowing experiences usually involved an injured horse and it's anxious owner. But there was a more dangerous species - the parents.

I was on the rail idly watching a night class once when the judge came over to me. He said, " Without pointing, watch as the horses go by, see if there's one with a white eye." I did, I could, and when he returned I indicated the white eyed horse which of course he had seen anyhow. I forgot about the incident. The judge pinned the horse down on the basis of the blind eye.

I was still on the rail when I saw out of the corner of my eye what appeared to be a group of agitated people on the secretary's stand surrounding the show manager who apparently in self defense suddenly pointed directly at me. They approached me. They surrounded me. They were angry. They were a corps of parents and assorted relatives. Apparently they had attacked the judge who blamed me, then marched to the manager to locate me. They surrounded me all talking at once. I gathered that their horse had been pinned at other shows in spite of his blind eye. In self defense the judge had blamed the show vet, and the manager to save his neck pointed me out. My first reaction was to place the onus back on the judge. But relying on courage I didn't know I had, I faced the gang of parents, aunts, uncles, cousins, the trainer and the rider who remained calm through it all. I tried to explain to them how a judge has a responsibility to consider any condition that may affect the safety of the rider or other riders. I wasn't having much success. The little rider hadn't said a word, so I extricated her from the rest to try to reason with her alone. She was becoming reconciled and understanding when the corps caught up with us again, with renewed energy. My situation was bordering on being dangerous when Mr. Crosbie, the show steward appeared. The show steward's role is to serve as a contact between the competitors and the management. He of course, should have been approached in the first place. Both the judge and the manager were remiss not to have told the protesters that proper show protocol was to approach the steward first with any questions or complaints. Mr. Crosbie listened to their tirade, relieving me from immediate danger. Then he explained to them how they could write their complaint to a proper committee including a fee which would be returned if the complaint was honored. But his final advice was what I believe is the most significant part of the story. He said, "Please wait five days before you write the letter." I realized afterwards that his advice was to allow time for passions to cool and reasoning to take over.

Another time, another show - "Doctor Mills -please report immediately to the Secretary's Booth!" No response. "Doctor Mills, you are wanted at the Secretary's Booth!" Dr. Mills was sound asleep in the back of his van. Putting in a full week's work, then getting up early to drive a horse van many miles qualified him for a stolen nap whenever possible. The van door swung open, "Dad wake up there's a horse having a fit!" I was led stumbling to the scene of action. The horse was indeed acting like an epileptic fit. He had been in the trailer when suddenly he went over backwards breaking his halter and falling out on to the ground in a seizure. I didn't have a full complement of medicine with me because I wasn't the designated 'show vet', I was just a vet at the show. I gave a tranquilizer which helped somewhat. Looking around the scene I noticed a bottle of tonic. One of the ingredients of the tonic was Nux Vomica. The active ingredient of Nux Vomica is Strychnine. This was interesting, so I asked the owner when he used the tonic. He said, "I dose him before a class to brighten up his performance. He's been sluggish to-day, so I gave him a double dose." This meant to me that the poor horse probably benefited from half a bottle. Winning is important sometimes. Strychnine is a tonic in appropriate doses. Inappropriate doses cause uninhibited stimulation of all the nerves in the body. I felt I was close to a diagnosis. The 'on call Show Vet' got there in time to give life saving antidotes. I had trouble finishing my nap and the horse missed his class, having been brightened up a bit too much.

JOHN LONG POLISH NAME

Our horse farm plus three daughters resulted in a steady procession of visiting young people. It's why I called it a Branch YMCA. If the hustle and bustle of the place displeased any of them they disappeared, if on the other hand they found it agreeable they attached themselves to a broom or a manure fork and stayed. In fact some stayed so long that it influenced their careers. I knew most of them by their first names, last names registered only after about six months.

There appeared at the farm one day a fine young Polish boy who eventually stayed long enough to get a job with Nancy in her hunter horse stable. He was a good kid. His name was John long Polish name. After a year he was still around so I decided it was time to learn his last name. It was a name with lots of connected consonants and syllables that I hadn't conquered thinking he might disappear and the effort would be unnecessary. This hadn't happened so I asked Nancy to write his last name down for me. I put the paper in my pocket. Whenever we met I would say, "Hello John," then pull out my note and slowly pronounce his last name. He laughed at this and so did I. Like I said, he was a good kid. After you pronounced it a few times it actually rolled off the tongue quite smoothly. John was more interested in the mechanics of the farm than the horses. He painted my 1938 Ford N tractor black with red fenders. He also kept it tuned up. John was a good kid, like I said.

FEELING GUILTY

The dog was a gentlemanly 10 year old hound in for his yearly check up with his long time client owner. We found him in good shape but his owner was a bit agitated. Seems she had been to a vet nearer her home apparently for the last time. He had treated the dog successfully, but before they left he asked her why she had never had the dog castrated. She didn't know how to answer that, so he went on about the social and pathological sins of not having it done. This confused her because the dog was in good shape and had never been any trouble related to his being intact. But the vet went on and on to the point that she felt like walking out. Obviously the well meaning advice had offended her.

This happens all too often, an owner comes in feeling good about doing nice things for his dog and goes out feeling guilty. He wanted to do what was reasonably essential to keep his dog healthy and had had a barrage of ancillary tests, vaccines and procedures thrown at him. This came as a surprise to him and was well beyond what his budget would allow. He goes out feeling guilty and resenting that the money he had spent was not enough. Furthermore he would be apt to skip the next yearly exam.

I have always made an effort to make office consultations as relaxed and pleasant as possible. This was as much for me as for the clients, but I did enjoy taking time to catch up on what they were doing and what kind of environment their pets were accustomed to. My wife often suggested that I spent too much time at this. My reply was that I was practicing Holistic Medicine by studying the whole animal including its life style, in other words by going beyond the itchy skin or the chronic ear in search of some environmental factors that could be contributing to its condition. To provide this relaxed atmosphere I have had a tendency to engage in simple little attempts at humor. One such attempt after retracting a cotton swab from deep in a dog's ear I have enjoyed the wide eyed surprise of a child by saying, "Oops - I went. too far, there's part of his brain". Or I have been know to say, "If you want the dog to be better, don't leave the thermometer in too long." Or I may confess that the best time for me to treat a sick animal is just before it is due to get better on its own, makes me look good. Often I am asked what kind of a dog their mongrel is. It's usually the result of so many generations of chance meetings in the street that I can't resist commenting, "What kind do you want?" These little peccadilloes sometimes got me into trouble, but usually they transformed apprehension into smiles. As a child, my first two experiences with vets were memorable because they were so unpleasant. It is important that little owners avoid an unpleasant first encounter. It's like cutting a nail too short on a puppy on the first visit. It imprints a permanent resentment that's sure to make the puppy become anti veterinarian.

I have always relied on word of mouth advertising, no spread in the Yellow Pages, no newspaper advertising, no garish road sign. I feel right about it, but it's probably been a trade off for my being non wealthy. It's my opinion that merchandising is degrading to the profession. Expense of education and over capitalizing on the physical plant often puts a practice under pressure to maximize every transaction and perhaps over-use the profession. I know of a vet who gets upset with his receptionist if the phone isn't ringing all the time. I believe that clients are more apt to remember the attitude of a receptionist than the hospital she works in.

ZOONOSIS

Zoonotic is the term for diseases capable of spreading from animals to humans. There are many of course, but I would like to write about two that I spent a lot of time with, - Brucellosis (Undulant Fever in humans) and Tuberculosis. These diseases can be spread to humans through cow's milk. Proper Pasteurization kills the disease causing bacteria in the milk. There has been State and Federal funding in an effort to eliminate these diseases from our cows for decades. Federally Accredited vets play a big part in this effort.

My first experience with country practice was riding with a Veterinarian in up state New York doing TB testing of dairy cows. The testing is done pre-dawn before the cows are turned out. It consist of a small interdermal injection of tuberculin. After three days the animals are examined. A significant swelling at the site of the injection indicates a reactor. The reactors are slaughtered and the farmer is reimbursed. This 'test and slaughter' method has reduced the incidence of TB to a fraction of 1%. Years later when on my own and doing TB testing I was shocked to pick up four reactors on my very first herd test. Years of testing after that I failed to detect a single reactor.

Brucellosis is controlled in the same manner as TB except that it is a blood test instead of a skin reaction test. Reactors are eliminated and the farmer is reimbursed.

A Brucellosis vaccination is given to calves between 4 and 5 months of age. It is an effective preventative, but the calves have a false positive reaction to the test for a time afterwards.

Sometimes in an outbreak of Brucellosis in a herd, we used to vaccinate the whole herd in an effort to control it. This of course made the cows test positive for a period of time. Which brings to mind my old farmer friend Henry Donaldson. Henry was a delightful old guy who had a twinkle in his eye and always delighted in poking fun at me. He did however, have the strange habit of preferring a shady deal to an honest one. It was much more fun for him. He once bragged to me about how he had bought a cow cheap because she was in poor condition. He then had her dehorned, fattened her up and sold back to the same man for double the price. That was relatively harmless compared to another one of his capers. It went like this - a week before his annual herd test for Brucellosis he got hold of some Brucella vaccine and vaccinated several of his cows whose value was less than their reimbursement value as reactors. They of course tested positive. He was paid his illicit money and old Henry had something to laugh himself to sleep with for years. If these capers weren't bad enough, he pulled one that crossed the line, why - because he pulled it on me. I had agreed to buy half of a fattened steer that he planned to have slaughtered for his own use. When the time came the packaged meat was delivered to me and I proudly presented a T-bone steak to our family kitchen. It was so tough that it destroyed my domestic tranquility for days. It must surely have come from an aged milk cow. I guess old Henry couldn't resist joking with me. My dog thought he had died and gone to heaven. He loved the stuff.

Henry is gone now, probably still chuckling about that deal somewhere. Gone also are most of the family dairy farms. I miss the warm barns in the winter, the sound of cows contentedly eating, the thousands of pre-dawn TB Testing, and yes the farmers, who were such a wonderful part of the New England scene, even old Henry.

WHO IS YOUR VET

Dorothy had Donkies, Mules and Arabian Horses, lots of them, I mean really lots of them. The purpose for all these animals was obscure. They were not groomed, halter broke, or trained. They were well fed and were quality animals, but failed to show it because of their rough appearance. She allowed several breedings a year that outnumbered the few sales. The population continued to grow. She was a delightful little gal who loved her charges but who seemed devoid of purpose for them. She used a small animal vet for her dog and a large animal vet for the horses. Neither of whom happened to be me. This was confusing to me since we were practically neighbors and I attended to both species. This all changed late one night when the door bell rang. My wife timidly opened the door to greet a policeman. His business turned out to be that one of Dorothy's mules had broken through the fence into the road and been struck by a car. The car must have had some speed because the mule had traversed the hood and smashed the windshield. The driver was remarkedly unhurt but not remarkably somewhat surprised by it all. He was most eager to leave the scene as soon as the mule was removed from his hood. The policeman seemed apologetic about disturbing us, but he felt he had to because Dorothy was hysterical and weepingly insisting that he do something, like get a vet, mainly me. He probably had to as a measure of self defense. My wife heard him mutter, "I think the mule is dead anyhow." We dutifully got dressed and made the call, and pronounced the animal deceased. She cried that the old mule had clocked hundreds of hours of trail riding in the past and this was an ignoble end for him. We agreed, commiserated with her, calmed her down as best we could, then went home to bed, wondering why she hadn't called for her own vet. This was the first and only call we had received from this good neighbor.

Now the plot thickened. The next day it so happened that a complaint was registered against Dorothy to the Society for Prevention of Cruelty to Animals (SPCA). Apparently someone thought she had too many animals to take proper care of. The SPCA officer arrived and his first question to her was, "Who is your vet?" Without hesitation my good neighbor replied. "Dr. Mills is my vet." Dr. Mills was her vet to the extent of one call to administer to a dead mule in the middle of the night. All that wasn't too bad except that Dr. Mills subsequently had to make several long non paid consultations with the SPCA Officers at her place. We urged her to cut down the population to a workable level to avoid prosecution, which she eventually did.

We managed to laugh about the whole situation even after she went straight back to her regular vet who had slept through the midnight tragedy. She was however a colorful gal who was always a pleasure to meet up with at the local diner. She was the only one who ever paid me with a winning lottery ticket, We remained good neighbors and friends.

MISGUIDED GOOD INTENTIONS

The owner was angry. "Was the other testicle normal?" he asked. "Yes," I said. "Then why the hell did you remove it?" "Gosh, I thought I was doing you a favor," I said. "What on earth do you want with an old donkey with one testicle? A gelding is much more useful". I began to think my good intentions were a mistake.

It happened like this - Joan was a compulsive animal 'care person.' If you were an animal with an incurable disability and were granted a choice of owners, Joan would be a good one. She had an old male cat that had difficulty urinating. She had an old horse that couldn't breath or chew and she had an old donkey who spent his whole life on Welfare except for the time he took part in a Christmas Pageant. Their recurring problems cost Joan lots of money but it's what she wanted to do. Her husband, on the other hand, disagreed with her wasting money on useless animals.

"Doc when can you examine my donkey?" it was Joan, "He has one testicle that is very large and growing fast!" Upon examining the donkey I was able to give her only one course of action - surgery to remove an enormous testicle. I was unable to predict whether it was inflammatory or tumor, but the prognosis was bad without surgery and only fair with it. The cost was discussed. "Shoot the thing," her husband growled. He had been lurking on the outskirts of the action in an unpleasant mood. "I'll have to let you know," Joan said. "I hate to lose him without trying, but as you can see I have a problem." The next day - "I'll pay you a little once a week and the rest when my Christmas Club comes due." A date was set.

The donkey was anesthetized and prepped for surgery. I made a bold incision into the melon sized tumor. Pus exploded out under pressure. "Good"' I said, "it's an abscess not cancer, we have a chance." The offending testicle was removed with some difficulty due to adhesions. I was on a roll now, so I thought, "Why don't I remove the other testicle. I could deliver a nice fat donkey gelding to Joan's husband at no extra cost. It might sweeten him up." Mistake!

The next day I stopped in to check on some bleeding and discharge. The following day I did the same. That's when the husband approached in an evil state of mind asking about the other testicle. He was unimpressed with my comments and followed us into the barn. "Are you going to charge me for these calls?" he yelled. Joan was now crying and the situation was tense. At this point I lost my customary cool and replied, "I hadn't planned to charge you, but now that you mention it, perhaps I will." Not being among the brave, I was looking for an avenue of escape, when he left. "I had no intention of charging you Joan, I drive right by every day and I'm genuinely interested in the donkey's recovery." " Well", she said, "it might be better if you don't stop in here for awhile. My husband is too upset." She didn't have to tell me that.

Joan paid me with her Christmas Club, the donkey recovered, and I regretted my misguided good intentions as I passed their house without stopping.

SNEAK ATTACK

Some cats have the strange habit of suddenly and unaccountably attacking the person who may be patting it at the time. Or they may ambush from behind a chair to attack one's ankles. The attack isn't entirely vicious and seldom draws blood but is a disagreeable habit and has been know to account for the change of address for many otherwise satisfactory cats.

Wonderbus became our Hospital cat by default. He was left with us for boarding, and was abandoned. In a case like that an animal can be disposed of after certain legal steps, but Wonderbus had a way about him and we never got around to the legal steps. He eventually gained freedom of the building and wandered around pretty much at will. Wonderbus did serve a purpose to some extent. The mice abhorred him and he actually would attack any cat that had escaped from confinement, thereby distracting the escapee until we could lay hands on it. He sometimes wandered into the reception room and functioned as an unofficial receptionist. Folks generally loved him. He had however, the 'sneak attack' habit that I previously described, not bad, but it was there, deep in his personality. Here's what banned him from the reception room - a large friendly client was waiting one day while I prepared some medicine for his dog. I heard this conversation, "What a nice cat, I'll pat you on my lap while I'm waiting for Doc." It was quiet, then I heard, - "Ouch, what jya do that for?" An apology was in order by the embarrassed vet. Wonderbus was accused of aggravated assault and banned from the reception room. Perhaps it is time for cat psychologists to enter the picture.

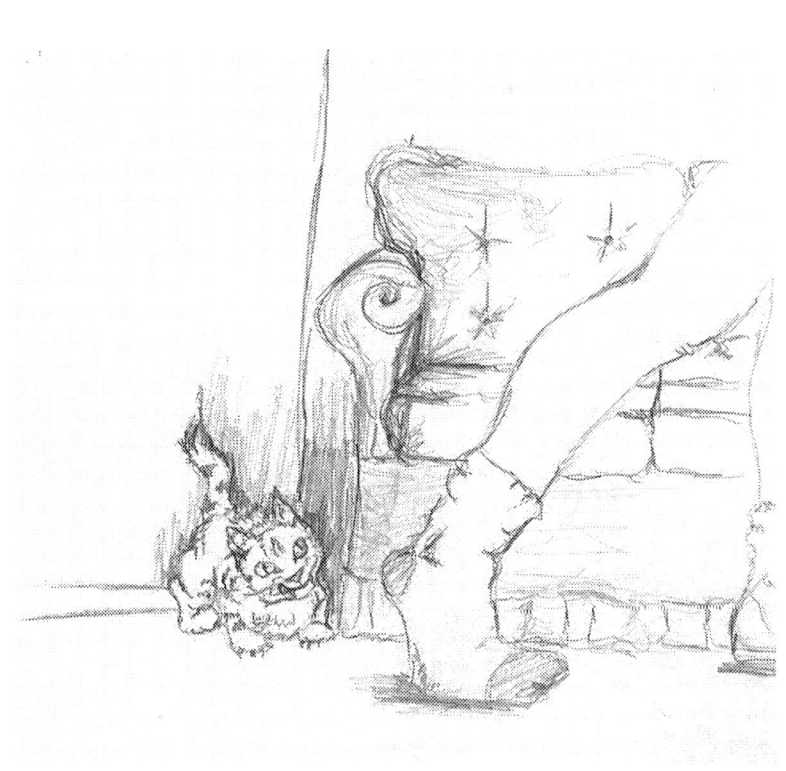

I'LL TAKE HIM

The big chestnut gelding was brought out of his stall. Jim said, "I'll take him!" The remark surprised and amused me. His attitude had completely about faced. It went like this.

Jim did stadium jumping, he was good at it although he had a lot of airborne time. He was tough and he loved the sport. His habit was to take a horse to it's full potential, then sell it and start over with a green horse, which is what took place this time. He sold a horse after it had chalked up an impressive record. This was fortunate for Jim but not for the new owner or the horse. Shortly thereafter the horse became sick half way over a jump and was dead upon landing.

In spite of this tragedy Jim now had the resources to look for another green jumper. He found one and I accompanied him to look over the new prospect, 'vet check' as they say. The conversation on the long trip was monotonously repetitive. Jim said over and over that before he would consider taking the horse home we would thoroughly examine him from the soles of his feet to the most distant parts of his body. He would longe him both ways of the ring, he would try him under saddle. He stated this over and over with set jaw and squinty eyes. He was determined to be very choosy. Shortly after we arrived at the stable, while I was groping for my stethoscope, the horse was brought out into the shed row for Jim's introduction.

Jim took one look at him. It was then that I heard his famous statement. "I'll take him!" - Resolve gone, the horse was loaded on to our trailer. I never had a chance to do my sensory, pulmonary, locomotive, cardio-vascular, skin, coat and suitability to the owner examination routine. I was shocked by Jim's sudden retreat from high resolve. But duly grateful to be relieved of my responsibilities. Actually the horse turned out to be fine. Perhaps buying on impulse ain't so bad after all.

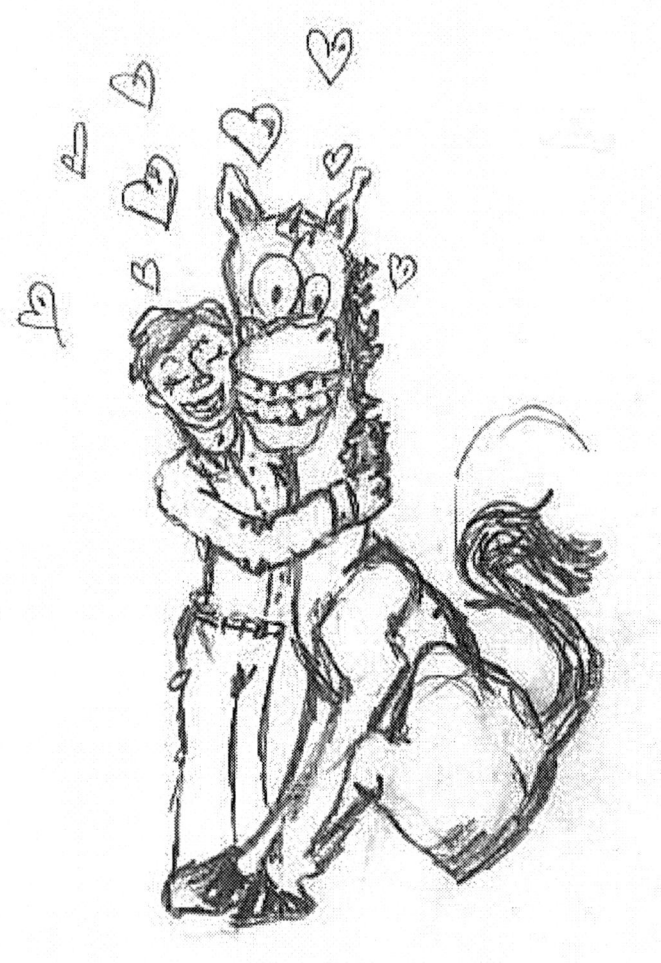

DISTEMPER

Like Milk Fever in cows the term Distemper in dogs and cats and horses is a misnomer. Distemper in dogs has nothing to do with their temper. It has a lot to do with their respiratory and nervous systems. It is seldom seen now, in fact many veterinarians have never seen a case of Distemper. It wasn't always like this. In the 40's and 50's Distemper was endemic in our area and throughout the state. It manifested itself mostly by a chronic low grade fever and by nervous symptoms. Case after case would present having suffered nerve damage and showing uncontrolled mouth motions with excessive drooling, commonly called 'chomping fits.' This frequently progressed throughout the body causing full body seizures. A very disheartening set of symptoms. In 74 cases of Distemper that I drew from my files I found that 28% of the 74 developed nervous symptoms, mainly facial twitching, chomping fits, seizures or chorea after recovery. Chorea can be described as uncontrolled rhythmical muscular contractions. 13% were euthanized, 27% died. It was a discouraging period to be practicing Veterinary Medicine. Subsequent improvements in the vaccines and more wide spread use of them have probably accounted for the rarity of the disease at this time. Since the disease is caused by a virus and has no specific treatment other than supportive care and antibiotics to control the secondary bacterial invaders, vaccination continues to be a valuable tool as a preventive measure.

Distemper in cats is also viral and causes an entirely different type of disease. The virus destroys all the white blood cells, leaving the cat susceptible to other infectious diseases. It is highly fatal if not treated to control dehydration and invasion of opportunistic bacteria. The vaccine is highly effective and durable and should be widely used

Distemper in horses likewise has nothing to do with the temper of the patient. The official name is 'Strangles.' It is caused by Streptococcus Equi. Being a bacterium instead of a virus, the disease usually responds to treatment. It is manifested by high fever followed by swollen lymph glands around the head especially between the lower jaws. These generally abscess and drain. It can spread rapidly through a stable to susceptible animals.

It appears that Distemper is a much used term that has little to do with the symptoms.

THE EYE OF THE HORSE

Instead of stepping neatly over the log the horse suddenly jumped up and leaped forward. It was at a 4H horse show. The little rider was thrown up only to come down hard into her saddle bounce a couple times and out of the ribbons. In the Trail Class at a Horse Show a cavelletti consists of some logs placed in the path of a horse to judge his ability to handle a similar obstruction on a real trail ride. It's a simple but meaningful test. The little competitor was embarrassed so she asked me afterwards how come her horse did such a foolish thing. "Well," I said, "it involves a unique aspect of your horse's eyes that I'd like to explain but it takes a little time. Why don't you invite me to talk about the eye of the horse at one of your 4H meetings?"

The invitation came and I accepted. I love to discuss the unique eye of the horse although I sometimes I feel the subject may be a bit too complicated for the younger audiences. It went something like this.

First of all let's remember that the horse has evolved over millions of years developing a body that has provided for his survival in the face of predators and changing environments. Other than the size of the horse man has done nothing to change this in the hundreds of years of domestication. It is therefore important to understand what we cannot change. In this case the eye.

To start with, your horse has the ability to see 360 degrees, a complete circle simply by a slight turn of his head, one way or the other. This is possible due to the fact that he has a combination of monocular and conjugated vision. Monocular - eyes that see to the side and individually. Conjugated - eyes that focus together and ahead, like ours. This was great for early survival but accounts for some strange behavior in his domesticated role. The horse has a triangular blind spot in front coming to a point at about half the length of his body when he looks foreword using his conjugated vision. This is because his eyes are placed on the far side of his face, not directly in front as ours are. He can overcome the blind spot simply by turning his head slightly, engaging one or the other eye to see ahead while obviously the other spans more to the rear. There is a blind spot in the rear as in front. Here again he can overcome this by a slight turn of the head. This gains a full rear view while the opposite eye scans where he is headed. What a beautifully designed system to survive a wolf pack chase. This is very important for survival in the wild, but accounts for some strange behavior in his domesticate occupation.

It's the blind spot in front that is interesting. For instance when you offer him an apple on your hand, it is usually knocked off. His sense of touch and smell tells him - apple - but the exact location is in his blind spot. While feeling with his lips, he usually puts the apple on the ground. This also explains the cavalletti experience. As he comes near to the center of the pole it is out of his sight, he can see the ends of the cavalletti but he has forgotten how high it is in the middle, so he over jumps in order to play it safe. With a little practice he will learn better concentration. By the same token, your hose does not see a pole directly in front of him as he takes a jump. He does it by memory. As a horse approaches a jump there is a point where he engages his conjugated 'two eyes ahead' vision. It is interesting to note that at this moment his ears are pointed directly ahead, coordinating with his eyes. He is now concentrating entirely on the jump. If his ears are pointed to the left or right he is interested in things to the side and he may refuse or fail the jump. Horses in harness are often provided with blinders to avoid their being distracted to the side.

Your horse helps to focus his vision by raising or lowering his head. His retina in the back of the eye has a flattened arc. If he raises his head, he sees distant objects clearly, and when he lowers his head he sees closer objects more clearly. Humans are able to change focus by changing the shape of the lens. Since a horse in the wild spends most of his time head down grazing, with a little imagination one can see how this capability allows the animal to see clearly the ground while at the same time scanning the distance for a clear shot at a Saber Toothed Tiger or a Mountain Lion. Here again his eyes worked fine when his business was to gather food and escape from predators, but at the same time accounts for some odd behavior in his present occupation. Many trail riders have had the experience of nearly flying over their horse's neck because he stopped suddenly and lowered his head to inspect a strange object on the trail, usually a simple shining puddle. He wanted to get that thing in focus, before he stepped on it so he lowered his head. Made sense to him, but nonsense to the rider.

Why does your horse have an oblong pupil, (the black hole in the center of the colored iris through which light passes to the lens) instead of a round one like ours? Remember his livelihood is to avoid capture. This means being able to scan around in all directions. To do this an oblong pupil is better than a round one, it enhances his peripheral vision. The round pupils better serve the chasers, not the chasees. The chasers' eyes are in front with conjugated vision, the better to concentrate on their prey. They don't need to see to the rear because they are not chased.

Why does your horse have a black mass, (Corpra Negri) on the upper border of his pupil? It's not know for sure. My theory is this. A grazing horse has dilated (opened wide) pupils because the ground is relatively darker. But remember he is also looking around the horizon for predators, an area with much more light that would have a damaging effect on the sensitive retina with the wide open pupils. Could it be that this black mass filters out damaging excessive light.

Have you noticed that when you sweep cobwebs above your horse's head he is disturbed? Since your horse has poor vision upwards, he instinctively may be fearful of a predator lurking above him. In this case a broom. Please don't forget that the physiology and instincts of your horse are very much the same as when he was entirely wild.

You can't see the prettiest part of your horse. Why? Because it's the retina deep inside the eye lining the back of the globe. Next time your Vet comes ask him to show you the retina using his opthalmascope. You will see a beautiful iridescent color, and if you persist you will see the optic disc which resembles a red setting sun.

So now you have an idea of why your horse:
- Over jumps a cavalletti
- Knocks the apple off your hand while trying to eat it.
- Cannot see the jump directly in front of him as he approaches it.
- Lowers his head and stops suddenly at a simple object in his path.
- Is upset at moving objects above his head.
- Has an oblong pupil.
- Has a black tumor like mass on the upper border of his pupil.
- Is sometimes obliged to wear blinders.
- Has a beauty undisplayed to the outside world.

By this time most of the 4 H-ers had lost interest beyond why a horse over jumps a cavalletti.

RIDING LESSONS

I stopped at the arena one night to watch the riding lessons. My daughter was instructing. As usual a few parents were also watching, some proudly, some anxiously. I asked one proud looking parent which rider he was particularly interested in. He was eager to point out his daughter and how well she was progressing and how she had a natural talent. I agreed with him and seized the opportunity to launch into my opinion of what learning riding skills can do for a child other than riding.. It went like this -"Learning to ride is a skill that is never forgotten. If riding is taken up again years later the skill will still be there, though some muscles may need tuning up. I said this from experience. Twenty years after playing polo at college I got on a horse at our farm and found the skills still intact. This is not to say that my riding was the precise and proper type taught by my daughters. But it allowed for proper rhythm with the horse, consideration for his mouth and back, and stay on him at all cost. But your daughter is doing more than just learning to ride a horse. For instance in the first lessons she showed considerable courage to mount a large strange animal. Then she learned coordination and rhythm, while strengthening her body. She will learn responsibility for a lesser being, including feeding, grooming, and general horse husbandry. At horse shows she will learn competition including winning and losing. Riding, showing, and having the responsibility for a lesser being may all help fill a vacuum that lead many young to waste time on the street. I used to tell my daughters that they can expect to win some classes they should have lost and lose some they should have won. If they show long enough it will average out. But in any case they should learn how to win humbly and lose graciously."

By now my new friend seemed a bit dismayed by my enthusiasm, but I hope he felt better about standing there in the cold arena watching his daughter learn all those things about riding other than riding. I didn't tell him that if his daughter continued in the horse game he might very well exchange his European vacation for her habit. He'd find out in time.

DOGS FOR HEALTH

The guy came into the exam room full of talk, and eager to tell me about himself and his dog. "My dog has taken 30 pounds off me and sent my blood pressure spiraling down." He came in for up-dating on his 'Almost Springer Spaniel'. The front part was a Spinger Spaniel, but his tail was long and had a fine display of long brown and white hair that clearly represented a few other breeds. The totality of which was a real fine dog. My interest in his remark encouraged him, so he went on. Incidentally, this is the sort of thing that prevents me from scheduling 15 minute office calls and accounts for our seldom eating lunch before 2 PM, but sometimes I feel it's my best contact with the outside world. He explained - "I've been a railroad engineer for many years, my run is a passenger train between Boston and Hartford. Through the years I have had a few suicides on the track. These were hard for me to take but earlier this year there was a tragedy that really got to me since it wasn't a suicide. I unavoidably killed two people who were riding on an all terrain vehicle. They were riding on the track. I came around a curve at 65 miles an hour, they were right in front of me. I hit the brakes and blew the horn, the girl looked back just as the engine ran into them. This effected me so badly that I was sent to a doctor. I was over weight and my blood pressure was off the scale. The doctor suggested that I get a dog and take long walks with him. I took his advice, got this dog at a pound, we went on long walks and it worked." I was tempted to mention a connection between a dog pound and an engineer's pound. But I didn't.

You see, I never would have heard this fascinating story if I hadn't allowed myself the time to listen. Three things impressed me. One - that he must have had a Holistic type doctor who took the time to study his patient's life style and suggest a change that might help. And two - that the Engineer took his advice. And three - a good dog can be a shield against the stresses in our society.

DO ANIMALS THINK

Some of the members of our discussion group claim that animals can think. I agreed with them as long as they put an upper limit on their type of thinking. My contention was so obvious that I think their's was influenced by a strong bias. In other words, I don't think they were thinking.

There are many observations of cases where animals think. I can name a few. Our Dachshund enjoys riding in both my wife's and my car. We occasionally leave at the same time. It is interesting to watch him stand between our two cars, his head turns one way and then the other. He is obviously trying to decide which way to go. He is thinking. Our dogs were confined in the kitchen one night when our deck caught on fire. The flames threatened the rest of the house. One dog said nothing, the other barked with increasing intensity until my wife investigated and saved the house. He was thinking, he knew something was wrong. Outside the fence of my chicken coop there is some grain on the ground. The door is opened. Some birds crowd the fence near the grain and fail to reach it. Others go away from the grain toward the opened gate and reach the grain. Are they thinking or are they using the trial and error method. Certainly some are smarter than others.

Dogs are able to realize many emotions identified with ours. Fear, hate, anger, envy, joy, love, and greed are a few. As we said, they also think - so why aren't they considered thinking animals? Why, because their thinking comes up short at the creative level.

For instance, since the earliest bonding with man, dogs have enjoyed the warmth of a fire. In all this time has anyone seen a dog put a log on a fire? Animals communicate by a wide variety of sounds and body language and use of their sense of smell and touch, but the communication is limited at these points. There is a wide gap in thinking between the highest non-human primates and the most backward of the human aboriginal societies. The top primate (man) gathers knowledge for new generations to build on, records history, appreciates humor, buries his dead, realizes his mortality, makes music, communicates with words, contemplates God, etc. These are the attributes of human primates and represent the type of thinking unavailable to our thinking animal friends. Individual animals can demonstrate unusual ability to think and they appear to gather knowledge over and above their peers. But the fact is that the gained knowledge is lost when the animal dies. The next generation must start from the bottom again.

My friends were hard to convince. Their love of animals blurred their 'thinking'.

From a dog's standpoint, what's so great about thinking. The dogs that I am familiar with, my own in particular, do just fine without it. He manages to have food, shelter, health care, love and his own personal chauffeur all provided on demand, If he could think he would probably have to do these things for himself.

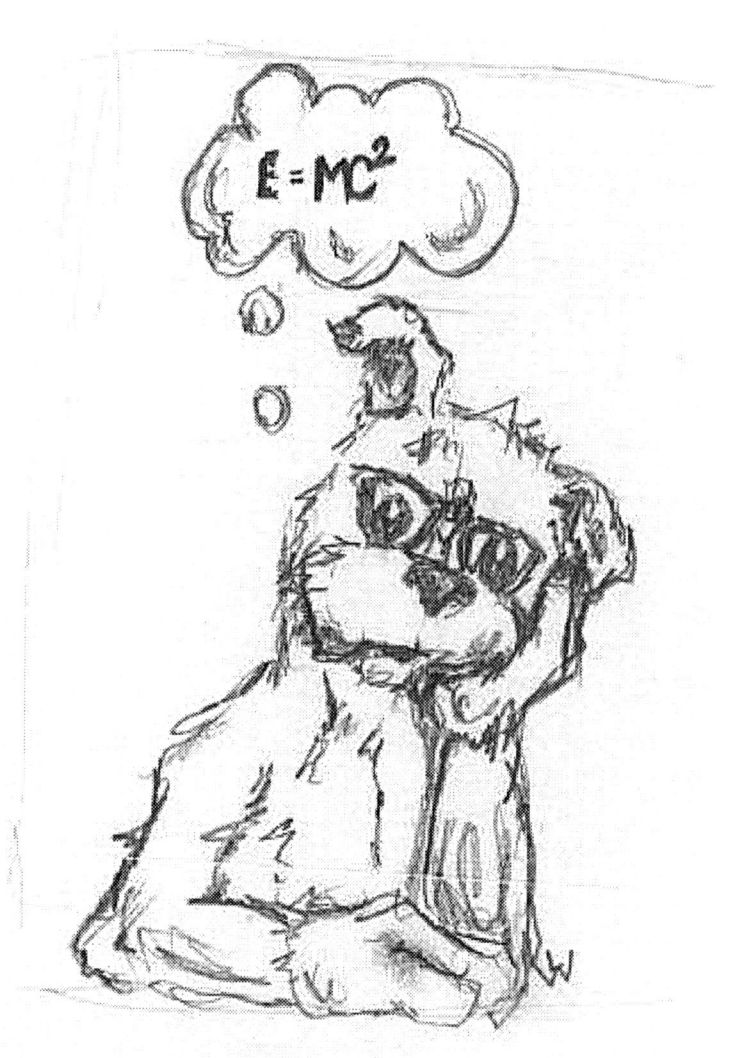

AGING A HORSE

Estimating a horse's age is often called 'aging.' him. It is challenging for both horseman and vets. Folks love to know how old their horse is, especially when considering a purchase. The teeth are generally used as an indication of the age. Up to five years of age the teeth are a reliable guide. This is because the permanent incisors (front row teeth) replace the deciduous (baby teeth) at a rather definite yearly rate. After five years of age one uses the surface of the incisors and the angle from which they protrude from the mandible and the upper jaw to 'age' the horse. There are cups (depressed dark areas) on the surface of the incisors that wear with time at a dependable rate. These are used rather safely to identify age up to eight or nine years. After that it becomes difficult to be sure. Experience is a big help, but it still remains an educated guess to be definite within three or four years.

I was often requested to tell the age of a horse. I considered myself to be rather good at it, and I became quite bold and adamant. Until,- one time. Sam asked. "How old is my daughter's horse, Doc?" I went through my routine of examining the teeth thoroughly. In all my wisdom I proclaimed, "She's ten years old, Sam." "Gosh Doc, we've had her twelve years." After that I always established how long they had had the horse before I ventured a statement. Generally after ten years, instead of being specific it is acceptable to just call the horse 'aged'. They are then as old as they feel and capable of performing.

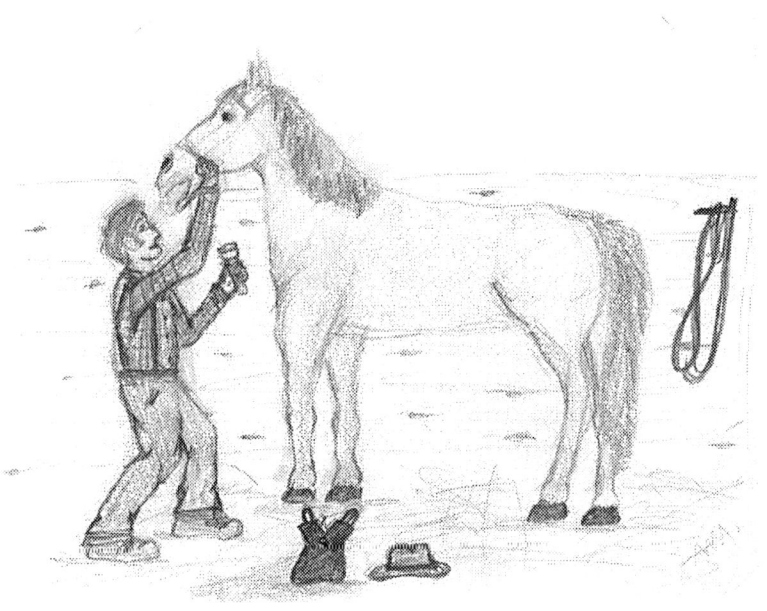

BAD TIMES – GOOD TIMES

Three daughters, horses, van, trailers, alarm clock and plenty of gasoline, these are the things of horse showing, which we did every week end for decades

Sunday morning, - dawn, - my daughter ahead driving the trailer with two horses. Me, I'm driving the van with three horses. We're due to be heading east to the show grounds. We go through the toll gate onto an access to the Interstate Highway. Immediately there is a divider, east to the right, west to the left, - simple enough. I am lighting my pipe, it helps me stay awake and alert. The van goes left, west. I see a horse trailer on the east bound access. Fellow horseman -"guess I'll wave to them." They don't wave back. Instead they are hitting their foreheads with their hands. "Strange people! - Oh my God, that's our trailer, I'm on the wrong access. I'm dead." There are horses in my van in the first class at the show. The next exit is 15 miles west. I panic, "I'll drop the horses at the next town and just keep going, they'll be sad when they miss me." I get hold of myself and try to figure a way out of my dilemma. I'm desperate. I remember a narrow grass medium ahead. My pipe has gone out. I'm alert now without it. I have a plan. I stop in the. emergency lane and wait until there are no cars in sight either way. I make a U turn across the grass medium on to the east bound lane and gun her. I can hear the horses thumping their feet as they adjust to the acceleration. Five miles down the road I spot a horse trailer in a gas station. I wave again to fellow horsemen. Again they don't wave back. This time instead of slapping their foreheads their mouths drop open. Peculiar people! I'm all set up at the show by the time they get there. "What took you so long?", I comment, which doesn't add to my already lowered popularity

I have a favorite word, -it's '<u>Dad</u>', I love to hear it. But a simple word like 'Dad' can have several meanings. First there is the regular, " Hi Dad". That's OK, like I said, I love to hear it. Then second there's, the louder more emphatic "Dad!", like - are you alive after falling off a horse. Third the rising emphasis going up the scale 'Dad of caution,' like on a dark night " Dad, is that you in there?" And fourth - there's the dreaded 'Dad' that starts with a higher pitch then fades downward. This clearly indicates disapproval, and probably has the most frequent use in my case..

We're on our way home after a show, we're tired, it's late. I'm driving the van. My daughter, the designated navigator is beside me. "Carolyn, do we take that left ahead?" "Right," she said. I turned right and it gets me the fourth type of 'Dad'. It takes three miles to find a turn around and there is very little conversation on the rest of the trip.

Sometimes things went right, but they don't make good stories. I got lost one night on the way home. My daughters and friends were asleep in various locations in the van. They were awakened by noises of boards, jacks and profanity. I had made a wrong turn and drove into a steep driveway to turn around. It was so steep that the rear tail guard contacted the tarmac. When I reversed, it dug in. Nothing moved after that, forward or back. It took a long time to jack it up to get boards under the wheels and apologize to the owner for the new dent in his driveway. I drove home with the fourth type 'Dad' ringing in my ears.

We stopped for gas on the way to a show one Sunday morning. I set the emergency brake. As we went up a hill from the station the cab filled with smoke. I pulled over and grabbed the fire extinguisher. In the side view mirror I saw about six kids eject air born from the loading door like parachuters out of a plane. I discovered the smoke was coming from the emergency brake that I had failed to release. I was barraged with the fourth type of 'Dad' from all six riders.

But the good times outnumbered the bad ones and as time went on they seem to have all turned into good times, and Dad is still my favorite word.

HEROICS

Eye surgery was clearly out of my line, but I had no choice. I was called to treat what appeared to be a routine inflammation of the eye. After examining the eye I dispensed my favorite eye ointment and was later disappointed when there was no improvement. A more thorough exam with an opthalmoscope revealed the problem to be a foreign object in the anterior chamber (clear area between the cornea and the iris).

The patient was a stylish Arabian colt. Being well fed and confined to a stall he had a lot of pent up energy that he sometimes expressed by climbing the stall walls. On one such occasion the trainer tried to discipline him by beating him about the head with a short whip. This was unfortunate because the end of the whip had some exposed fiber-glass strands. One of the blows struck the colt in the eye. A piece of the fiber penetrated the cornea and broke off. Hence the foreign object.

At that time there were few places for referral of surgical cases and they were hundreds of miles away. Most cases had to be tackled in the field. This was one of them.

The colt was put under anesthesia on the floor of my arena. The cornea was opened and I was able to retrieve the piece of fiber. The lids were sewn shut for a supportive bandage. The eye healed and the horse went on to win high awards throughout New England. Apparently the judges didn't notice that the eye was a bit smaller than its mate. The colt's vision was not affected.

The floor of an arena is no place to attempt sterile surgery. In those days improvisation bordering on heroics played a large role in our activities. It meant operating on the grass or on an arena floor down on a level with the patient. It was kneel down bend over work. Currently horses are lifted up on surgical tables which are far more comfortable for horse and doctor and allow far more complicated and successful procedures. This is better for all concerned, but some of the challenge and excitement disappears when a case is referred for others to resolve the problem. Progress often has some pain.

THUNDER STRUCK

I went hunting with a friend who was eager to try out his new German Short Haired Pointer. The dog had been quite pricey and my friend had great expectations from him as a bird dog. We finally flushed a Pheasant, my friend fired and missed the bird whereupon we also missed the dog. He had ejected in terror at the sound of the shot. "My God, he's gun shy!" my friend yelled. I had to restrain him from shooting the dog when we found him cowering under a bush. A gun shy hunting dog is a complete failure at his designated job. Instead of jumping with joy at the sight of the shot gun being lifted from the gun rack, he trembles and hides. He won't be a hunting dog. In fact he may be less than satisfactory as a pet since he is probably scared of all loud noises and particularly thunder.

Thunder is a source of abject terror for a surprising number of dogs. A client asked me why that was, while picking up some tranquilizers for his thunder struck dog. "I had to pay for repairs on my neighbor's screen door," he said. "He burst through his screen door and hid under the guy's bed during a storm." I was sorry he asked that question because I had to admit I didn't know the answer. I believe they are born with the phobia, which is strange since canines evolved in the environment of thunder storms. Since it might be genetic, it behooves one to be careful not to buy a pup from scary parents. The explanation of these abnormal fears probably belongs to dog psychologists. I do know that it is practically impossible to break a dog away from the fear.

Speaking of unfortunate behavior, one can't help wonder why your clean, neat miss perfect little lap dog does on occasion take delight in rolling in the most foul smelling rotten stuff there is. Then this little character well trained in etiquette comes into the living room as proud as can be, only to be dunked into the tub.

I do have a theory on this. Could it be that there is an instinctive action here? Fleas are brainless ubiquitous pests that have a good sense of smell. They are not interested in jumping on a dead animal, there being no blood to feed on. In fact they are eager to leave a dead animal. So a dog that smells like a dead animal may be protecting himself from the aggravating visitors.

DECAPITATION

There's no doubt that the local doughnut shop is a great generator of anecdotes on life. It happened this way. As usual I sat at one end of the counter to catch up on the Vet journals. Presently this guy came in and sat close by. He looked vaguely familiar, he was well seasoned or should I say many seasoned. I could identify with that, and he glanced at me a couple times so I ventured a "Good morning." He said, "How did you bruise your hand?" It was obvious that he was more interested in my hand than me. "It doesn't take much," I said, "I take a lot of aspirin so my capillaries bleed easily." "My brother has the same problem,"' he said, "You touch him and he turns blue." By now I was curious to know this guy's name. I hated to ask, so I got cute. "What's your brother's name?" "Arthur," he said. That didn't help much so I gave up. "Arthur who?". "Menard," he said. That did it, the name connected, as did some memories. I exclaimed. "For heavin's sake I used to vet your cows, in the 50's and 60's, remember?" He had been retired from dairying for perhaps 30 years, but he claimed he remembered. I guess he did because he mentioned a severe dystocia (difficult birth) that had occurred on his farm,-and we reminisced.

It went like this. Incidentally I should warn you that this might be an unpleasant subject for some. You may do well to turn the page to the next story. We recalled that on this dawn Ray had found one of his cows exhausted from trying to give birth during the night. He woke me up with his problem, and I set out eagerly because I actually enjoyed that type of case. They appealed to me because it involved mechanics more than infectious or organic disease. The patients were in life threatening discomfort and with any luck could be relieved with one call. This case was a bit unusual. The calf's head was presented to the outside world not accompanied by its front legs. When the legs are mal positioned backward the shoulders remain too large to allow the body to advance through the birth canal and the calf cannot be born. This calf had died and the head was swollen. Normally the head can be retracted back into the body of the uterus to allow enough room so the legs can be advanced foreword into the vagina, thereby lining up with the head for an acceptable birth position. This is done by attaching an obstetrical chain to the fetlock of the calf (just above the foot) then pushing the body of the calf back into the uterus while an assistant with moderate traction pulls the leg foreword. It works great and is fun to do. This one was different. The head could not be returned because of its swollen condition and the body could not be advanced because the shoulders were too big.

There was no way to reach the mal positioned legs to advance the delivery. A virtual road block in both directions. The head was the problem. It had to go. With proper tools including a wire saw We removed the head from the body. Having done this the body of the calf was readily pushed back into the uterus and the legs pulled foreword as described, and the calf was delivered. The cow breathed a sigh of relief and started to eat. Ray went in for his breakfast, I got mine at a diner. The cow went on line in a couple of days. Decapitating the dead calf was unsavory, but all other parties were grateful.

Back at the doughnut shop Ray and I were glad to renew our acquaintance. He commented that I had done a great job to save his cow thirty years ago and he was grateful - grateful but not enough to buy my coffee.

NO RETIREMENT

Some varmint had the indiscretion to savagely tear apart all of all my client's ducks - except one. This victim had the skin removed from his neck and the bottom part of his oesophagus opened to the outside world. When he took in food, it reappeared through this hole. In spite of his infirmaries Duck chirped quite cheerfully. My first remark was that there was no chance. Perforated Oesophaguses are notoriously difficult to deal with because of the constant movement and fluids that interfere with the healing process. But then I thought, maybe ducks are different. I sadly remembered the case where I had opened a horse's oesphagus suspecting an impaled wire foreign body. It failed to heal and the animal had to be put down. But that was a horse - this was a duck. Let's see what happens.. Ducks and chickens have minimal sensation in their skin. My tech held the beak while I pulled the rift together with suture material, the patient objecting more to restraint than the operation. The following day Duck was able to drink without water extruding it from the rent - good sign - but not yet conclusive. We fed Duck Rice Crispies soaked in water which was eaten greedily and swallowed with some difficulty. Duck went home and we awaited the outcome.

At a coffee break a week later a guy next to me said, "You're Doc Mills aren't you?" I replied in the affirmative, reluctantly taking the risk of being reminded that I had put his pet to sleep when he was 10 years old or somthing. Not this time - "You took good care of my sister's duck, he's swimming around and doing fine." This cheered me up when I needed it.. Even though it wasn't exactly open heart surgery, success is welcomed in all sizes.

I frequently find myself groping for a response to the, "When are you going to retire?" question. I usually stumble around with some inadequate remark like, "A body in motion tends to stay in motion." But since the duck affair I have a better answer, - "If I was retired, how could I have taken care of this guy's sister's duck?"

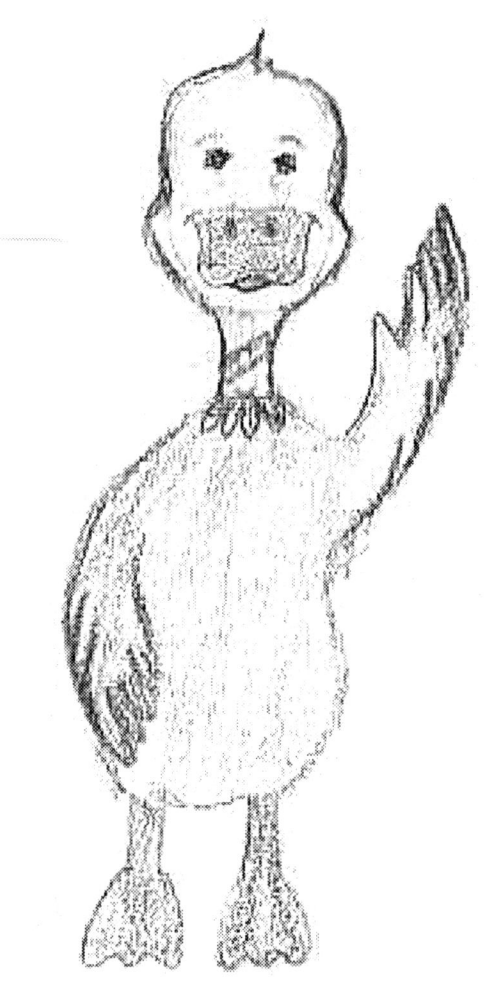

THE POTENT GELDINGS

Horse auctions have traditionally been an avenue of escape for the owner of an unwanted or unsalable animal. People who buy at an auction do so in hope of getting a good animal cheap. They are fully aware that they may go away with a bargain or a disappointment.

"Doc, I've got an embarrassing problem with a gelding I just bought at an auction." I expected him to say that the horse came up lame after the bute (horse aspirin) wore off. This unfair act is sometimes done by a seller so a horse will go sound temporarily in order to expedite a sale. But no, he said, "I put him in with my other horses and he proceeded to breed my mare." Understanding his embarrassment, I still had to ask him, "Did he actually have an erection and penetrate the mare?" "Yes", he said, "I'm positive, very positive."

After examining the problem I agreed with him, amazed because his horse appeared to be a gelding. I explained to him that geldings sometimes are sexually attentive to mares but fall short of the complete act. "There's a good chance that he's a ridgling", I said, "a ridgling is a partially castrated stallion with one testicle remaining in the abdominal cavity."

I went on to explain that in the new born both testicles are in the abdominal cavity. They descend into the scrotum later. Occasionally one or both fail to make the downward passage through the inguinal canal. These retained glands are unable to produce viable sperm, but they do produce testosterone. A horse with one retained and one descended testicle can reproduce. If both are retained, the animal can breed but not reproduce. On rare occasions a Veterinarian for reasons best known to himself, will unfortunately fall short by removing a descended testicle and leaving the abdominal one in place. Removing the undescended testicle requires an abdominal opening which calls for a great deal more preparation. Which may be why it is on occasion not done. However it should be done because horses in this condition are undesirable and are often passed from owner to owner eventually ending up in an auction. Having been bought 'as is' at the auction my client couldn't return it and he liked the animal, so he agreed to an exploratory operation.

With my daughter as the anesthetist we prepped the animal and I made an ample incision into the abdomen. With gloved arm I reached in and was fortunate enough to quickly pick up an erratic testicle and remove it. Intuition told me to go back and look for another. This resulted in the removal of the second one. Instead of the half castrated ridgling that I suspected it was a cryptorchid (two undescended testicles). We looked at each other in wide eyed amazement, then put the brand new gelding back together.

The owner's remark when told about the operation has always stuck with me. He said, "I know when you buy a horse at an auction, you take what you get, but <u>enough is enough</u>!"

This reminds me of a similar situation that occurred following another gelding operation that we did. The horse was sold shortly thereafter and he soon began to cover mares in a very convincing way. The new owners were not happy and sued the sellers for misrepresentation of the goods. I was contacted by a lawyer in regard to the surgery. He asked, "Did you leave an undescended testicle in the abdomen?" Feeling a bit stung by the question, I said, "No, they were both available and I can count to two." The horse was sold again, same thing happened. Lawyer called, same question, same answer.

When asked for an explanation, I hypothesized that since the adrenal gland has three zones, one of which produces a small amount of sex hormones perhaps this zone was hyperactive on the testosterone side, causing all the trouble. Whatever the cause I insisted that I could count to two.

WHEN TO RETIRE

I isolated myself at the end of the bar in a donut shop as I often do in order to catch up on a little Veterinary Journal reading - when my privacy was broken. "Hi Doc, how are you?", the old man asked. "I'm fine thanks, how are you?" I dutifully replied. "Fine," he said. Platitudes over; then he asked,-- "Do you remember me?" "Oh sure" I said, hoping he would take it at face value. No such luck. "Then what's my name?" he persisted. Not happy with being trapped in a falsehood, I said, "You know who you are, so why are you asking me?" Luckily that crack didn't offend him and he went on to say that he was the mechanic who worked on my car twenty years ago. At that point I really did remember him and we had a good nostalgic conversation." Are you still working?", I asked. "Oh no, I retired at 61." "So what are you doing with your time?" I asked. "Absolutely nothing, I'm 77 years old." This confused me because I was pushing 82. years and still working, so I vowed to lie when he asked me my age. I didn't want to belittle him in any way or perhaps I just wanted to avoid his 'what kind of a nut are you' look. He didn't ask me. He left. I went back to reading and wondering which of us was right.

VIGNETTES

Good Morning, what's on the agenda for today?" "You have two calls to go on this afternoon when you get done with the hospital work," my early morning person said. That sounded reasonable enough and the morning progressed without a hitch. There were a few phone calls. When the work was done and I was preparing to go on the calls my tech said, "You don't have to go." "How come?". "One died and the other got better on its own," she said. "Wow", I said, "That's two of the worst scenarios that can happen to a vet." That set back gave me a chance to reiterate once again something that I never noticed in the text books, Mainly that the best time to treat a patient is just before it's about to recover on it's own. Makes you look good.

- - - - - - - - - - - - -

At home nursing an upset stomach I answered the phone." My horse has colic bad, can you come up and take a look at him?" It was the dreaded night time call. I didn't recognize the voice and groped for a way to let some younger vet earn his keep on this winter night. So I asked, "Are you a client?" "Oh yes", he said, "You took care of my cow when she had milk fever." Still not recognizing the voice, I asked, "When?" "About thirty years ago", he said. That shook me up so much that I decided to respond, to the call, wondering whose colic was worse, the horse's or mine.

Since we had somewhat the same symptoms the horse and I took Bicarbonate of Soda on a 'one for you and one for me' basis. Between the medication and the exercise both the horse and I began to feel better. I assume that the horse continued to recover because I never heard to the contrary. Perhaps he was waiting another thirty years. I guess that qualifies him as a client.

- - - - - - - - - - - -

At a coffee break I happened to run into a fellow horseman. While discussing mutual problems we compared various ways of manure disposal. I said that I spread manure on the pastures. He did too, he said, then added that it was also good to spread on potatoes. I added, "To each his own, but I prefer gravy on mine."

- - - - - - - - - - -

"Put this medicine in his ear daily until there's improvement. But you should understand that your dog has an inherited tendency toward the ear condition. We can treat the condition, but I doubt we can treat the tendency. After improvement, you should be alert for a return of the symptoms. You may want to apply the medicine once a week to keep the condition from returning. However, we'll play it by ear." "OK", the owner said as he left, "By the way, was the pun intended?"

- - - - - - - - - - -

There should be a course in college called 'Unusual Cases' and how to handle them. For example - The harried phone call went like this, "I'm supposed to be taking care of my neighbor's cats for the week end, but she left the wrong key. I can't get into the house. Do you think the cats can live until Tues.?" I told her I was sure they could and not to worry. When I told my Tech about the dilemma she commented, "Check the gold fish."

- - - - - - - - - - -

He was the biggest dog in the world. Big as a brown bear. He lived next door to our dog hospital and often lumbered over to pay us a visit. From time to time his owner entered him in the hospital for maintenance work on his ears or updating. When we were done with him we would attach a note and a bill to his collar and push him out the front door. He would dependably return home repaired and bearing the messages.

- - - - - - - - - - -

As he left with his old dog friend I reminded him, saying, "This Rabies shot is good for three years." He thought a minute and then said, "If he doesn't live beyond two years is there a one third refund?" Appreciating his creative frugality, I said that I would apply the credit to his next dog.

DON'T TOUCH ME

I always extolled the virtues of a general practice but sometimes it becomes a bit too general. To-day we had a one pound rat, a 10 pound rooster and a one pound Umbrella cockatoo hopefully to put on the road to better health. The cockatoo was a juvenile that refused to advance from hand feeding to self feeding as would be expected in the wild natural state, as a result it was quite thin but seemed healthy. He was white with a hint of yellow in proper light. His crest and tail feathers were absolutely beautiful. I casually asked the owner how much one would expect to pay for a bird like that, She said, "I paid 1400 dollars for this one." "Then what are you letting me touch it for?" I said.

EMOTIONS AND COLIC

A colicky horse creates all kinds of emotions. There is pain and fear in the horse. There is compassion, anxiety and often sadness for the patient's human friends. This is a story that illustrates my observation about colic and human emotions. It may be extreme, but it's based on fact.

There was a time when our Morgan mare foaled a perfect colt. Shortly afterwards the mare developed colic and died on the surgery table. We raised the colt by hand and with the help of a surrogate dam who adopted the foal after her foal had been weaned. We called the colt 'Bogie'. The colt grew, was gelded and became a beautiful animal. My daughter Carolyn, took Bogie to Florida where she gave lessons on him and. consistently won in Trail and Morgan Hunt Seat Classes. Given his history with us and his success at whatever tasks he was asked to do, Bogie became loved and cherished by all who knew him.

Bogie got sick. He was found one morning exhausted and in great pain. What follows is not so much about Bogie's sickness as it is about the human emotions related to it. He failed to respond to initial treatments so Carolyn trailered him fifty miles to an Equine Surgical Hospital. After the surgery Bogie's expected recovery was disappointing and a few days later it appeared necessary to undertake a second operation. It was a difficult decision for Carolyn, but she is of a disposition that stays the course and takes all risks necessary to save her animals. She has a strong rapport and emotional attachment with them, Bogie in particular. She and her husband John, drove the many miles many times to do what they could to help, only to see Bogie fail to eat and grow weaker day by day. They were devastated. Finally they were given the sad news from the hospital that Bogie would not live. They gave up hope and stopped their visits. That sets the stage.

Two days later the doctor, who had practically worked her heart out on the case, called John to say that Bogie had not died but was showing faint signs of recovery. John's emotion, other than that of happy disbelief was cautious. "Doctor", he said, "under no circumstances do I want you to tell this to my wife. If she gets her hopes up only to be dashed again, it may be more than she can take and I doubt I will be able to live with her.'" Mum" became the word. Carolyn assumed she had lost her horse and went into mourning. She began to receive condolence cards. This state of affairs lasted for five days.

John received another phone call, "John we are pleased to be able to report that Bogie has started to eat, if this continues we expect him to recover." Joy - then panic! - He thought, "How can I tell my wife,- she will be furious that I let her think Bogie was gone all this time. I've got to think of a way to give her the good news and save my neck at the same time." Where his neck is concerned, John is quite resourceful.

This was his strategy. He convinced Carolyn to meet him at the ranch where Bogie had been stabled. This was difficult because Carolyn wasn't anxious to go back to the place where Bogie took sick, but she went. He wrote the news on a note and left it on the seat of his car. At the ranch, surrounded by friends for protection, he told her to read the note. The emotions that ensued were great, one of which turned out not to be anger after all. He had misjudged her understanding, and emotions of joy were the rule.

Bogie recovered after a few set backs that were treatable and went back on line. It is interesting to note that Bogie's life started with a tragic failed effort to save his dam. Years later when his turn of fate came, he was saved. There may be many reasons for the different outcome, but one of them I am sure was the emotion Carolyn and John felt for Bogie that expressed itself in extraordinary perseverance, sacrifice and nurturing love.

MAY YOU HAVE A LONG LIFE

Roland was perhaps a decade beyond his first Social Security check. He weighed about 120 pounds. His Great Dane weighed a little more. Roland liked me, his Great Dane didn't, in fact he hated me. Dane became down right dangerous at the mere thought of me. He had previously created a despicable scene in the exam room when he chased everybody around in fear. Roland weight for weight was no match for Dane whose adrenaline level must have approached his blood volume. Most of the folks in the adjacent waiting room, hearing the confusion, had the discretion to exit their pets to safety. When the beast lunged at me with teeth bared I, in self defense, pushed a chair between us, missed and hit Roland in the knee cap. Roland, trying to restrain the dog was too busy to complain about his knee. When ,the battle was over, I gave this advice. "Hereafter leave him in the van, we'll deal with him there."

Eventually the time came to see Dane again and he was left in the van as requested. As I approached the van in the parking lot, it literally rocked as Dane charged from seat to seat. I was relieved that Roland didn't take him out as I had visions of them both disappearing over the horizon, with little old Roland bouncing around on the end of the leash. I usually tried to doctor the dog over the phone, wracking my brain so he wouldn't have to be brought in. This day things were no better, perhaps worse. He needed his yearly shots. There was no way to avoid his coming. I loaded three syringes, gave one to Roland and asked him to get in the van to give the shots himself. Dane was not compliant at all, he leaped from seat to seat rocking the van like a series of speed bumps might do. It was obvious that Roland couldn't give the shot unless I distracted the dog. So I stood outside the driver's window to accomplish the distraction. The driver's window was partly open. Dane charged his drooling head out the window furious to the point of biting the side view mirror apparently mistaking my reflection for the real thing. But Roland was determined. The plan worked and Dane got his shots, one at a time, although I nearly lost my hand when I handed the syringes through the window.

    Relaxing in my office afterwards, Roland wiped the sweat off his brow and became quite talkative. He wanted to know if he now qualified for a license to practice. Then he launched into a remarkable story. It went like this. He said that a State Cop remarked to him that he had a very protective dog. Roland agreed, but how did the cop happen to be aware of it. The cop said that he was the one who entered Roland's house to help move him to the hospital. He is diabetic and since his wife died he had not been careful with his diet. He was passed out in his home for two days before he was discovered. The police had to enlist the help of the Dog Officer before they could remove my friend to a hospital. Having told me all this, Roland went on to say that since that episode he had put aside some money to take care of Dane if he (Roland) should pass away. With the money was instructions to submit Dane to my care while seeking a new owner. The prospect of Dane being submitted to my tender loving care stunned me and I wished Roland a long long life.

SWAMP FEVER

In the early 1970's we became aware in the horse population of a disease characterized by weakness, anemia, swelling of various parts and often ending fatally. Earlier there had been 75 deaths at Rockingham Park in New Hampshire. It was found to be caused by a virus and spread by contaminated hypodermic needles and vectors such as mosquitoes and horse flies. It was described as Equine Infectious Anemia (EIA), commonly called Swamp Fever. The disease has a dormant or non-sick infected stage in which case the horse can live a comparatively normal life. However under conditions of stress, fatigue, sickness or exposure the virus can become active, multiply in the blood and bring on the symptoms of the active disease. No treatment or vaccine has been developed. The only means of control of the disease is by isolation or destruction of infected animals, a course of action greatly resented by many, especially owners of non-sick carriers. All of which leads up to the most tragic day of my equine practice career.

At first the only way to make a diagnosis was to inject blood from the suspect into a sacrifice pony, followed by checking the temperature three times a day. A significant rise in temperature of the pony was considered a probable diagnosis of EIA. This was an unpleasant procedure and detected only the actively sick horses. It became critical to be able to detect the dormant non-sick carriers as well as the acute cases. This was ultimately done by Dr. Leroy Coggins at Cornell University. It was accurate in detecting antibodies to the virus, indicating either a dormant or acute stage of the disease. It became known as the Coggims test and is still widely used.

Since there is no treatment or preventive vaccine, many states have adopted a law calling for quarantine or sacrifice of reactors. This resembles the 'test and slaughter' method of eliminating TB and Brucellosis in cattle that has been done for many decades. It should be mentioned here that the 'test and slaughter' method used in cattle is different from the 'test and quarantine or sacrifice' method used in horses for two reasons. One -there is compensation for lost cows from Federal and State funding. There is none for horses since there is no public health involvement. Two -the loss of a horse is not only financial but as a companion animal is often met with severe emotional stress.

Terry Thomas ran a stable about twenty five miles from my office. He boarded horses and ran supervised trail rides. He was a client and friend for many years. Being in a low profit business he had to be frugal in buying replacement horses. He bought a number of horses at an auction. Horses imported across state lines were required to be tested for EIA. This was hard to enforce It was also required to periodically test all commercial stables, and all horses entered in shows or any equine event. It came time to test Terry's stable.

I drew the blood in a routine way, sent them to the lab, and forgot about it. Three days later I received a harried phone call from the Division of Animal Health. "Did you draw the blood at the Thomas stable properly?" "Of course I did, why do you ask?" "Why, because there are thirteen reactors," he exclaimed. "What, that's hard to believe, they appeared so healthy," I said. " You've got thirteen reactors, we want them all re-tested and if they repeat they all have to be destroyed according to the law." I was shocked and wondered if they suspected that in order to save time I had drawn thirteen samples from one horse and picked the wrong horse. The same horses were positive on the re-test. Apparently they were known positives that were shipped into the State illegally to be sold through the auction market and had escaped the mandatory testing. The massacre reluctantly became my responsibility. When the dreaded day came Mr. Thomas led the condemned animals out one by one for the sad euthanasia. They were buried in three massive graves. It took Mr. Thomas years to recover from the loss. I have always been pleased to be part of any disease eradication program but this particular effort has left me with a feeling of guilt. There were so many of them and they looked so healthy. The stable was tested again one month later. There was one more reactor, then no more. In the interim Terry showed up at my hospital with a very sick horse in his trailer, it was barely able to stand up, obviously nearing death. Hoping I could perform a miracle, he started to unload the patient. Fortunately I was able to stop him. I knew there would be no miracle from me and I was reluctant to have a dead horse in my parking lot. The poor animal died on the way back, suffering from the final stages of the disease. It appeared we had missed him in the testing.

As I mentioned previously, the control measures were severely resented by many horse owners. Not unexpectedly, it was eventually tested in court by a man who refused to comply with the destruction order of his non-sick positive reactor horse. I was called as a witness for the State because of the experience with the Thomas Stable. The State won the case and EIA control law prevailed. EIA is a small threat today but calls for continued surveillance to head off any recurrence of the epidemic.

Such were the difficult early days of Infectious Equine Anemia.

VENGEFUL SKUNK

Wild animals as pets are a bad idea. Although they are cute at first they often become a burden and are eventually neglected. If released back into the wild they are no longer able to survive.

We used to descent skunks, not often and not willingly. My first experience at the job was as an intern. It was also the most memorable. My boss had given me the job and dispatched us to an open field for obvious reasons. The skunk was put into an ether box. This was a box with a glass front so the patient could be observed. Ether was administered through a hole in the top until the animal appeared to be anesthetized. In this case the appearance was deceiving. I removed the skunk and started the surgery which was immediately resented. The little guy was only partially under, 'light' as they say. At this moment my boss appeared on the scene to check up on me. The worst happened. I can see it now. A perfect shot of skunk scent arching through the air zeroing in on my boss's trousers. My apologies fell on deaf ears. It was the first time I realized the guy had no sense of humor.

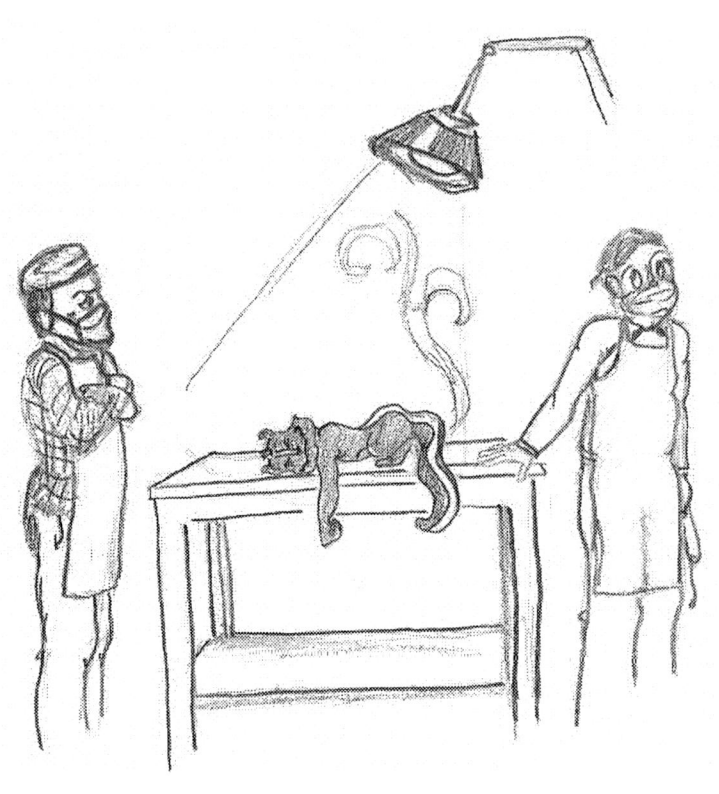

ANIMAL RIGHTS

In most advanced societies today, Human Rights are a big issue and include the rights of minorities, mentally handicapped and felons, this while the idea of Rights of Animals generally wait in line.

Recently, however, Animal Rights have moved up the line and are realizing more attention. There have been many attempts to define 'Rights' of Animals. For the most part, they tend to become complicated and confusing. The definition put forth by the Humane Society of United States seems more straightforward and clear than most. It emphasizes that there are Legal and there are Moral Rights of animals.

Legal Rights are clearly defined and represented by Federal laws such as the Animal Welfare Act, the Endangered Species Protection Act, and a law preventing soreing of American Saddle Horses which applies to the practice of irritating the fetlocks of performing horses to encourage a higher front leg action deemed useful in the ring.

Moral Rights are less clearly defined, but applicable to many more situations. In general, the Moral concept defines Animal Rights to be as near Human Rights as possible. Put simply, when an Animal Rights situation arises it calls for weighing the suffering and deprivation of the Animal against the comfort and gain realized by the Human, then honoring the decision. Obviously, there has to be some reality in all this. Personally, I have zero regard for the rights of rats. On the other hand, when weasels killed my Banty Hens, I trapped them and relocated then, with the admonition to apply the their animal rights to their natural prey. When my wife catches a fly in her hand, she releases it outside, but a mosquito gets short shrift. Most of us make no connection with the killing of a cow when we order a steak. Actually, we are the predator at this time. We are simply delegating the killing to someone else. Are the cow's rights abused in this case? By applying the Moral concept here of weighing the loss of one against the gain of the other, we can possibly justify the sad act of slaughtering. From the <u>Human</u> Rights point of view, this appears to be justified. The 'food chain' of all animal life was evolved long before Humans gave thought to Animal Rights, and remains necessary for the survival of countless species of animals.

What can be considered some of the general abuses of Rights applicable to animals? Consider the Right to develop its natural potentials in an environment where it is best suited; consider the right not to be subjected to unnatural physical or emotional stresses; consider that whoever confines an animal is Morally responsible to provide the creature necessities that it has been deprived of the ability to provide for itself. Consider the Right of a species not to be driven to extinction. Surely here Moral Judgment of the loss of one against the gain of another weighs on the side of Animal Rights.

What can be considered some specific abuses of Animal Rights? Consider the extreme method of confinement in raising pigs and veal calves, allowing room only to get up and down while denying all other creature comforts; consider starving chickens to force a moult, consider amputating Sharks' dorsal fin for Oriental soup, leaving the Shark to die. Consider the killing of Elephants for the illegal Ivory trade, leaving the huge body to rot; consider killing the Rhinoceros solely for their horns to enhance the Arabian Libido. (I tried it while in Kenya-It doesn't work!) Surely Moral Code weighs in on the side of Animal Rights in these cases.

Rhinoceros horn trade is decimating the species, but is also in my opinion, senseless. The Ivory Trade, on the other hand, is based on demand for a valuable product. It has been shown that the best way to save the Elephants is to make it profitable for them to be alive for the Safari tours. There is no profit in viewing a rotting Elephant from a Land Rover. On the other hand, Ivory is a valuable product and should be a national resource. I am among those who believe that the Ivory should be harvested by trained wardens, taking specific, non-breeding, old Elephants for the ivory and meat. This would have little affect on the total population. It would, however, discourage Elephants form becoming too tolerant of close human contact which results in their encroachment onto farm lands as totally unhunted animals are prone to do.

Back home, Animal Rightists object to activities such as tail docking and ear trimming of dogs, declawing cats, etc. They believe that an animal should not be subject to pain to satisfy the whims of their owners. Others believe that since the surgery is done under anesthesia, a day or two of discomfort is a good trade off for a life time of loving care. Weighing the pain of the procedure against the increased value as a pet engages the Moral code of Rights.

As far as ear trimming is concerned, it deals with a much earlier whim that brought about pendulous ears through hundreds of years of selective breeding. There is not one species in the wild that has pendulous ears, not the canine, feline, equine, bovine, or rodent. The Elephants' ears are supported more vertically. Their big floppy ears are used as a cooling device and to display curiosity or aggression. Please understand that I am not advocating ear trimming. It is just that if one elects to have it done, there should be no guilt feeling. We have a little Dachshund with adorable pendulous ears and a big Boxer with admirable erect ears.

It appears that certain Breeds of dogs may be considered to be programmed cripples. What do I mean by that? I refer for example, to an English Bull Dog, so short nosed that he never takes a normal breath and so bow legged that he cannot trot, much less run; or a Poodle so Poodely that hair grows in his ear canals; or a Pug dog so Pugsy that he snores when he's awake; or a Sharpei with facial skin folds so loose that his eyelids roll inward, allowing his eye lashes to contact the cornea, possibly causing blindness if not corrected, etc., etc. Using Morality to define Animal Rights in these situations would seem to come down heavily on the side of the life long pain and discomfort of the animal exceeding the whim and pleasure of the human. I have long contended that these breeds could maintain their identifying characteristics without going to such crippling extremes. A Basset owner recently told me about a Basset party she had taken her dog to at which they had a contest among the many Bassets. I asked what the contest involved. She said, "We measure for the longest ears and the least distance from chest to ground." These are two of the crippling aberrations that Bassets are programmed to live with. I once treated a Basset that had fallen down stairs after tripping over his ears. I refrained from negative comments with difficulty. Dog show judges with an Animal Rights point of view could be a positive influence in this direction.

In the developed countries, there are encouraging efforts to recognize Animal Rights on an ecological scale by reestablishing animals into their natural environment. Wild Turkeys are prospering in our Eastern Woods, Wolves are back in some National Parks, dams that interrupt Salmon runs are being selectively opened. Animal Rights are on the move now, and we hope for the future. Do not confuse this with pure altruism on the part of Humans. We have come to realize that we are part of an all encompassing ecology on which Humans are eternally dependent.

While acknowledging the all encompassing ecology, we should at the same time recognize that there is a great separation between Humans and Animals. To seek a fair relationship with the lower Animals, their Rights should follow Human Rights, as much as Morality and Reality will allow. There are many examples of the goal of a fair relationship between man and the lower animals.

<u>Reality</u> is that food animals must be sacrificed.
<u>Morality</u> is the act of improving the well being of these animals in all respects.
<u>Reality</u> is that world wide humans are encroaching on wild life habitat.

<u>Morality</u> is the preservation of wild life habitat.
<u>Reality</u> it that humans are the top preadator.
<u>Morality</u> is how to fit Animal Rights into the <u>reality</u>.

It is fascinating to contemplate the chronology of the various phases of Human Animal relationships from the beginning to the present. In the earliest days of evolution, humans were prey of such animals as the large felines and canines. Then humans invented spears and group hunting and changed their role to that of predator. Then, in time, they became masters of the beasts of burden. During all this period the Rights of Animals were the furthest from their minds. The earlier relationships are gradually fading as new ones take over. Now predation of animals for food by man is mainly sport, except for a few aboriginal societies, (slaughtering of domestic animals has replaced it.) And now we see certain species of animals as valued companions, while other wild species are protected. It's true humans are now occasionally eaten by predators, and there are still beasts of burden, but these have become a rarity. Now we see Human Animal relationships evolving towards Rights of Animals and preservation of species. It has been a long ride for man from being the hunted to being the steward of all of the animals.

UP TO DATE RABIES

The door ringers were very upset. "Can you please loan us a cat carrier?" It seems they had hit a cat down the road, it was badly injured and they wanted to bring it to us for help. We loaned her the carrier. It wasn't long before they reappeared at the door, carrier in hand, no cat. They said the cat was convulsing and they were afraid to approach it. Would we go after it. Leslie, our general practitioner assistant volunteered to go with me. The poor cat was in extreme convulsions as reported, making it dangerous to rescue. While I was trying to think of a text book way to deposit the victim safely (for me) in carrier, Leslie not being burdened with college learning and more resourceful, got the job done. My role was degraded to holding the carrier. Whose cat was it? We looked for a collar, Leslie found it. A Rabies tag number from our Rabies Clinic gave us the information. The cat remarkably recovered from a concussion. The owners have become grateful to us henceforth.

An important link in this chain of events was the Rabies tag, illustrating a collateral advantage of the all important vaccination. Many lost pets are returned through the number on their Rabies tag. Rabies vaccination is immensely important to your cat other than returning it home. It is one of the most effective vaccinations. If a human is bitten by a cat, it is important to know the cat's vaccination record. If your cat is bitten by another animal, it is important to know that the biter is Rabies vaccinated. In the too often situation when your cat comes home with a bite wound, the aggressor is unknown and the cat wont squeal on it. There is no way of affirming the vaccination status of the aggressor. A cat with up to date vaccination is protected, thereby avoiding a six month wait to be sure of its non Rabies status. It is as important to protect cats from Rabies as it is dogs.

TORSION OF THE UTERUS

Kay entered her barn at dawn and immediately realized something was wrong. Good horsemen can sense a problem just walking by a stall. In this case her five month pregnant Morgan mare was lying down instead of calling for hay. She got up, but refused to eat and continually looked at her side. Could it be the dreaded colic?

My phone rang. She described the symptoms. "Can you come?", she said. "Yes", I said, "but first give her my favorite colic remedy, walk her a bit and let me know." I turned over in bed, but sleep wouldn't come. I knew she'd be calling back, so I was ready when the second call came. "Ok I'm on my way."

The little Morgan failed to respond to initial medications. The rectal exam was next. My sleeved arm passed over the rim of the pelvis searching for the offending intestine. The pregnant uterus was encountered first and following the uterus my arm was turned clockwise. To my surprise there was a torsion (twist) of the uterus. This is rare in horses, but rather common in the bovine in late pregnancy (described in another segment). The diagnosis was quickly changed from colic to the real problem. My first reaction was, "Why didn't I stick with small animal medicine, I could be peacefully vaccinating a cat or something?"

This was in the days when you either 'do it yourself or it don't get done.' Our first attempt to correct the twist used the Newtonian law of physics - 'a body in motion tends to stay in motion.' We led the mare down a steep bank at a brisk pace, then stopped her suddenly, hoping the momentum on the fetus would rotate it back into position. Nope. Next we transported her to a local arena. There she was cast and rolled in the opposite direction of the twist, hoping that as she came to an abrupt stop the momentum would reverse the twist. Nope. The next day she was still in distress. Surgery was the last hope. She was brought to the utility room of my small animal hospital. Following sedation, clipping the hair, and cleansing the area, I gave local anesthesia and made a standing approach into the abdomen. With my arm in a sterile sleeve I reached in over the uterus and rolled the little fellow back to its normal position.

While suturing the incision I thought, "If this works, maybe large animal work ain't so bad after all." It worked and the mare went on to foal in a normal manner.

In college we are taught the basics of surgery. It is impossible for every student to perform every type of surgery. Many challenges of surgery are met with the trepidation of first time case. The greater the fear and anxiety the greater the feeling of satisfaction if all goes well. This was one of them.

SPEEDY DACHSHUND

Our newly acquired Dachshund pup surprised me with his speed which was nearly as fast as our Boxer's who was obviously much bigger. So I watched. It soon became apparent to me that the Dachshund's reputation for having a long back is not deserved. His shallow body and short legs simply give that impression. Given a normal depth of body and length of leg, his back would no longer appear to be abnormally long. Then how does he go so fast? Here's how - when he goes at the gallop he greatly flexes upward his lower back (lumbar) vertebrae then rapidly extends them to propel himself foreword in coordination with the action of his hind legs. These two actions propel him foreword at a speed that belies the length of his legs. At the gallop the Dachshund's back is noticeably arched far more than the Boxer's. At the trot there is very little flexion of the lumbar vertebrae with either dog. This intense use of his lumbar vertebrae for propulsion may be a contributing factor to the high incidence of disc failure in the Dachshund. Given normal depth of body and length of leg, the back would not be relatively long and thereby not so stressed. This action which is normal for rodents like Weasels and Ferrets may not be good for our little short legged friends who got that way by selective breeding over many years to enable them to be effective Badger hounds, reversing the evolutionary plan of Nature.

BUT DOC -

"But Doc you're on the wrong end of the cow." I could understand the dairyman's concern because his cow was very lame in her hind foot and I was working on the front end of the cow giving an intra venous injection into the Jugular vein in her neck. The condition she was suffering from had the rather unsavory name of 'foot rot.' It was a severe infection that caused swelling between the cloven hooves, pain, lameness and a marked drop in milk production. It was a cause of grave concern for any dairyman. In the forties and fifties the treatment was labor intensive and the cure was less than satisfactory, often leaving a scared deformed foot. Treatment involved hoisting the rear leg up with rope in order to clean, medicate and bandage the area. The medicine was strong stuff like copper sulfate and strong iodine. The effort was resented by the cow and had to be repeated several times. The problem was that the infection was deep seated and our treatment was on the surface.

Then came the treatment mode that attacked from the inside instead of the outside. It was an intravenous injection of a sulfa drug far from the disease area and accounted for the initial skepticism. Skepticism that quickly turned to appreciation. It became one of the most dramatic and predictable therapies in veterinary medicine at the time. The cow would feel better and put weight on the foot within a very few days. Gone was the cowboy type rope and bandage treatment.

GRANDPARENTS

It has been noted by the media lately how much grandparents are being involved in raising their grand children. This is obviously a good thing when it becomes necessary and it recalls to my mind a similar instance but with an equine grandparent or more properly, grand dam.

The dam and new born foal were doing fine. The foal was gaining weight and strength daily. The owners decided to breed the mare back on her second heat period. The dam and foal were shipped to a stud farm at the proper time which is where the tragedy happened. The mare panicked while on a cross tie. She pulled back, the halter broke and she fell forcefully over backward. She never got up. Her spinal chord was interrupted in the cervical region.

The foal was returned home and put in a box stall with her grand dam and the owners began to hand feed her with substitute milk. The foal, of course, continually nuzzled on the mare's dry mammary glands, hoping for nutrition from a warm live nipple instead of from a bloodless rubber one. Which brings us up to the point of the episode. For whatever reason, be it maternal instinct or substitute hormones that came into play urged on by the situation, the grand dam came into her milk and successfully raised the foal until it was weaned. Kudos to grandparents in all species.

HOT TIP

Companion and show horses occupied most of our doctoring time. Racing Thoroughbreds were seldom seen. The Thoroughbreds we did see were the ones too smart to run fast so they ended up as Hunters. However we did see a few racing Thoroughbreds, mostly for R&R at our stable. Occasionally we had one in for treatment. The horse responsible for this story was one of them. During his therapy it became necessary for him to return to the track. In order to continue his treatment we agreed to visit him at the track stables, which sets the stage for this little experience.

At the track the treatment was done and we had a moment to look around. The horse's trainer was present and he was apparently eager to return the favor of our visit to the track to treat his charge. He drew us aside and whispered a hot tip for the next race. He said that No.5 was a sure thing, it was his turn. My daughter and I fortified with the inside information showed up at a betting window and laid down impressive bets on No.5 to win, acting like sophisticated insiders.

"And they're off!" No. 5 stayed with the pack through the back stretch and was improving his position with every stride. His odds were very good. We were practically counting our money. But on the home stretch our dreams and I'm sure the jockey's and the owners' and No.5's were suddenly dashed. Our horse suddenly dropped to a walk, the jockey dismounted and led his horse over the finish line. We looked at each other speechless and then started laughing at ourselves, sophistication destroyed. On the return trip, in retrospect after making fun of our being so naive our attitude changed to concern for the horse. It's a tough game of self sacrifice.

IT WAS WORTH IT

It was 8 AM when a thoroughbred stable called in to request help with a colic case. This was twenty five years ago. I happened to pull out the record of the case while poking through the archives. Let me repeat the chain of events. It might be useful to some young reader contemplating a career in Veterinary Large Animals by helping him or her to become aware of some of the possibilities involved.

That morning was December cold and the roads were December icy. The stable was at the top of a hill. Three feet from the top the truck slid to a stop. Nothing to do but back down. Three feet from the top was as useless as half way up. Next time I generated a reckless rate of speed before I hit the bottom of the hill. Same thing. The exigency plan was to circumvent the hill and approach the place from the opposite direction. This worked but took another hour and ruined any chance of my keeping a dentist appointment. The horse apparently suffered from a colon impaction (lower bowel constipation.) I administered to the patient and left expecting him to improve. At 11 PM that night however, the horse relapsed and the stable called for further help. I responded, as I did at 2 AM, as I did at 8 AM the following morning, then late again the next night. This was during 10 degree weather. I am pleased to report that the horse recovered, which of course makes it all worth it. It should be realized that some fail to recover in spite of all heroic efforts. I don't wish to discourage any aspiring youth, I merely want to apprise them of some of the surprises. Stick to your dream.

INSURANCE SALESMAN

While on vacation from college in the late thirties and riding with a vet for the experience, I ran into one of the surprises typical of this profession.

The order was to castrate a stallion. My mentor decided to attempt the surgery on the standing animal. This kind of spooked me, but the procedure proceeded nonetheless. He started by injecting the area to be operated on with local anesthesia. This may have anesthetized the area, but it surely made the patient leery of any future approach to the area. I was handed a twitch to apply to the victim's nose.

Nose twitch applied, held firmly with trepidation. Surgeon reached between hind legs, surgeon made cut. Horse reared up, horse flung front leg above twitch arm, leg came down on arm with vengeance. Twitch flew one way, assistant flew second way, horse chose third way, straight out of barn. Horse in evil state of mind.

I uprighted myself, brushed off some bedding, and checked for wounds. My first thoughts were about a change in career, perhaps to selling accident insurance to veterinary assistants.

Let me hasten to say that such a bad scene would not happen today and for a long time previous. Scientific research has provided us with sedatives and anesthesias that allow immensely better techniques.

I have often thought there should be a short course in college describing the way it was fifty years ago. It would help students to appreciate the medicines they are privileged to use.

IN SUPPORT OF GENERAL PRACTICE

If any readers are interested in Veterinary Medicine and are searching for the proper field to go into, you might be interested in the following article, which obviously is my choice.

My interning years were spent with general practitioners so it was natural and fortunate for me to follow in their footsteps. The life style has been good to me and I encourage young vets to consider it. Very few do. I have failed to impress them with what in my opinion a general practice can provide in self-satisfaction and enduring interest.

Somewhere in the sixties many dairy farms disappeared. The gap was soon filled by the companion horse. The winter warmth of the dairy barn was traded for the cold of a two or three horse stable. Most of us adapted readily if not eagerly to the changing environment. The patients and owners were different but the country practice was still the same.

Leaving the acknowledged stresses of a small animal hospital for the open road is like entering a new world, a world of changing seasons, fresh air, different types of people and animals. It provides the advantage of variety and altered challenges. It staves off burn out and boredom. A recent survey noted that horse owners appreciated a vet than can also treat their dogs.

A general practitioner can handle a large percentage of all cases. Referrals are easy and appropriate.

Realizing that all people are not equally comfortable with all types of animals I encourage a mixed practice for those who are. They will be more apt to enjoy their work into their later years.

WINNIE

On the third time around the ring she lowered her head, planted her front feet and sent her rider flying out of the saddle. The mare was University of Connecticut Winsome, known as Winnie, the rider was I, known as Dad.

My wife and three daughters were new farmers and newer horse people. We were considering Winnie as a foundation mare for the farm and a show horse for the young riders. Winnie apparently disliked out intentions for her future and decided to send us packing by bucking me off. Which she did. But Winnie's plans failed. I got up, dusted myself off and said, "Well take her." At that point, unbeknownst to us, we had matriculated into Winnie's School of Horsemanship.

We had spent the day looking at disappointing Morgan prospects until at our last stop we were shown Winnie. She was beautiful, made more so by contrast. Instead of the typical Morgan short back and rounded rump she had a long back that carried out to her tail head. Her eyes were set wide and framed by a beautiful face. Compared to the other poorly groomed, rather rough looking horses we had been shown she immediately impressed us. We were interested, so my daughter volunteered me to try her under saddle. At this point in our equine experience I was the designated rider, an honor destined to be short lived. There were eager pupils in the wings.

"Winnie, Winnie, Winnie, why were you such a harsh teacher? Did you have a mean or impish streak in you? I prefer the latter. Was it that impish streak that sent me out of the saddle? We were neophytes, you were young and we all had a lot to learn. When you joined our horsey group your impish streak came with you. Your habit of divesting yourself of your rider on impulse didn't end with our first encounter. In your new home you tried it a number of times until eventually I'd had enough of this impish streak. This time you tried it when I was having a bad day. I managed to bump back into the saddle and with strength I didn't know I had and with complete disregard for Animal Rights, swung a right hook to your ear. My daughter claims your ear hung down for a week. You never did it again, which is perhaps the point of my telling about it. We were both teachable. The teacher often learns best by teaching. You were teaching me how to stay aboard an impish mare and I was teaching you some equine manners. There followed a series of misadventures with you that became learning experiences for both of us. Do you remember the time when we got out of the sleigh you were pulling to walk beside it because the snow had melted in the road ahead? You suddenly trotted off with the sleigh threatening to leave us all behind and certainly to wreck the sleigh. I got you under control only by leaping on to the back runners and reining you in with all my strength. Lesson well learned by teacher and her students. Then there was the time you refused to go foreword over a bridge, preferring to back my buggie over the bank instead. You had been over the bridge under saddle many times before so it was hard to believe you were just being cautious. We were at an impass, you were stubborn and I was frustrated. The more I urged you foreword, the more you backed. I got out of the buggy at the edge of the river bank and holding your bridle I backed you and the buggy over the bridge. Perhaps it was a lucky stroke of reverse psychology. If backing was your way of protesting, Winnie you were invited to back. After that mutual learning experience you walked properly over all bridges. While I'm on the subject, I'm sure you remember when you had a panic attack in the trailer on the way to a show. You leaned into one side of the trailer while trying to climb the partition. It was a frightening experience for all of us. We had to off load you in the middle of Main Street. We moved the partition over a little, reloaded you and somewhat shaken continued the trip. You had taught us something about trailering horses. We got to the show late but unscathed. These were all grade school lessons, the high school lesson was soon to follow. This lesson is perhaps best described by my daughter who at the time was sunning herself on a high point overlooking the pasture."

"Winnie, Winner, Winnie – why were you such a harsh teacher? I saw Dad bring you out in harness and surprisingly hitch you to the heavy buck board wagon instead of the buggy. I went back to sleep with one eye open and witnessed a scene which opened both eyes and matched any of Hollywood's wild west creations." Winnie was used to a light buggy and when she was clucked foreword, she immediately resented the heavy buck board. She showed her resentment by doing exactly the opposite. She backed up and Dad was losing control fast. Both my eyes were open now but I began to wonder if I was having a bad dream. "Winnie, Winnie, Winnie, why did your school test us so hard in so many ways? Perhaps you hoped we would fail the tests and give up." Dad by this time had lost all control of his aggravated mare and when the wagon began to impact his fence, he also lost all control of his temper. In order to reverse Winnie's direction and save his fence, he slapped her rump soundly with the end of the reins. My bad dream had turned into reality and both eyes were eager to take in all of the action. With the slap on her rump Winnie overreacted and reversed her direction immediately. In fact she leaped foreword into the traces so smartly that one of them broke, and then the fun began.

The wagon now being pulled by only one trace, angled sharply, sending one of the shafts between her legs. This completely unraveled her, so she no doubt responding to her instinct of survival by speed, set off at a full gallop wagon in tow. My Dad, on the other hand responding to his instinct for survival by any means, jumped off the wagon. He brought the reins with him and tried to pull wild Winnie in. Instead of that she circled, which left Dad in the middle while she maintained full speed at the end of the long reins. This lasted for a surprising length of time while the shaft was bouncing back and forth between her legs. At first look one might have thought that Dad was longing the horse and wagon. Which he wasn't.

My daughter, sensing disaster, leaped to the scene to try to restore order. Winnie listened to her and came to a trembling halt. Her legs were abraded but not lacerated. We hooked her to the buggy before she could develop a mind set against being harnessed. She performed with perfect decorum, although our faint hearts failed to ask her to back up. There were other lessons after the buck board fiasco, but they paled by comparison and are therefore hardly worth mentioning. We eventually graduated from her school to become what could be called qualified horsemen.

By now we had come to realize that other than Winnie's singular conformation, she also had instincts, emotions and intelligence that would be most useful if we could funnel into a show horse personality.

After the graduation, our oldest daughter began her showing career on Winnie. They went through many many shows on many many week ends when their ribbons were scarce and insignificant. During this time we learned how our habit could easily represent a European vacation and how alarm clocks and gasoline were essential equipment. The three girls on their respective horses provided the losers necessary for the winners to be winners. That all changed suddenly at a three day show that was a traditional gathering of the local clan. It was combined with a county fair with all its noises and strange animal smells, not to mention that a misguided parachutist had chose the show ring for a landing spot. Winnie paid more attention to the county fair than to her business at hand and was particularly unnoticed for three days. On the final day we were making plans for a departure and I was talking horses and politics with some local natives when over the loud speaker came, "And the blue ribbon goes to Carolyn Mills on UC Winsome." This snapped us to attention. It qualified them for the evening championship classes and completely preempted our plans for an early departure. The night class found our extended family on the rail. It was now dark out, minimizing the county fair distractions. Winnie was all business. The judge saw a small rider properly attired and in perfect synchrony with a large graceful horse, skillfully making solo passes by the judge. Winnie was taking her aids with perfection. The selection was obvious. "And the blue ribbon goes to Carolyn Mills on UC Winsome." From the threw me on the third time around the ring, through lessons, to this championship ribbon had been a long many set backs but not without its share of fun. Their victory pass was worth all the harsh lessons Winnie had put us through. It was a synergistic example of the sum of the little rider on Winnie being greater than the sum of the little rider on another horse or the sum of Winnie with another rider. This ended their 'also ran' competition days. It started them on years of winning up and down the Easter Seaboard. Winnie's School had paid off. She became our week end warrior who made us famous. She was admired and envied by many. She was ridden by a little girl who after many many horse show week ends was suddenly a young woman who had been Winnie's best pupil. Over time Winnie gave us two great foals. She was continuing to teach us when without warning an intestinal stoppage took her life. She is buried in her school yard pasture and will be remembered as long as memory lasts.

ATTITUDE

The client asks, "What kind of a dog is he?" It's a question that is frequently put to vets when the proud owner presents his dog for examination. The owner is of course hoping for an opinion that reflects his desire for his dog to be a breed that it most closely resembles. The vet is often tempted to 'give em what they want to hear.' It does no harm to have the owner leave happy. In my own case if the guy seems to be broad minded, I have been known to remark, "Your dog is the offspring of a pure bred coincidence." Then I try to make amends by explaining that the most important part of a dog is his attitude. One should start with the attitude and build a dog around it. If a funny looking mixed breed dog has an attitude that brings warmth and companionship instead of aggravation and disappointment to the household it will be a successful pet no matter what its breed is. Then if my broad minded client's mind is still broad, I go on. "Let's talk about this companionship vs aggravation factor that constitutes a dog's attitude. For instance – does the dog respect his house breaking training or does he eliminate whenever it pleases him? Does a dog consider every stranger an enemy until proven different or is everybody a friend until proven different? Does your dog trash your house when you leave him alone or does he guard the house and greet you with enthusiastic love when you return? These habits have more to do with natural attitude than breed. While I had his attention I went on. Next in importance to his attitude is your attitude, can you adapt to his physical characteristics. Remember that big dogs need big space and big exercise. Long haired dogs shed long hair and must be groomed frequently to avoid unsightly matted knots and they tend to bring the outside inside with them. Dogs with pushed in noses tend to have protruding lower jaws, difficult breathing and may have persistent stains under the eyes. I don't mean to denigrate any type of dog. But I do mean to encourage prospective owners to anticipate what comes with them. By now the owner was eager to get on with the examination of his mixed breed dog and sorry he brought up the subject in the first place.

In fact since I wasn't able to identify the breed of his dog to his satisfaction, he parted with what I considered a rather bad 'attitude.'

STAY OF EXECUTION

Veterinary doctors have a unique ability that human doctors do not have. They can euthanize a patient and it can be done for any reason. Performing euthanasia is a <u>privilege</u> when the patient is suffering from a disease or infirmities of old age to the point of destroying its quality of life and often decreasing the quality of life of its owners. Euthanasia becomes an <u>obligation</u> when the animal is physically healthy, but it must be done because of an aggressive dangerous irreversible attitude. When euthanasia is requested for reasons other than disease, age or attitude, the procedure becomes a <u>moral dilemma</u>. There probably isn't a veterinarian in the country who hasn't kept these unfortunate animals in order to try to place them in a home. On one occasion that habit back fired on me. In the early uninitiated days of my practice a cat was brought in to be disposed of because it had become an inconvenience for the owner. My fee was paid and I postponed the moral dilemma. In the interim my tech asked if she could adopt the cat. Eager to avoid a moral dilemma, I foolishly agreed and she gave it a good home. In spite of this the cat had the indiscretion to make its way back to the home where its inconvenience had made cause for its demise. Whereupon the owner wanted to include me in the killing spree. He made it necessary for me to explain my larcenous behavior to the board of registration. My penance was to pay back my fee and expedite the moral dilemma post haste. Which I did. I obviously should have had permission for my misguided kindness beforehand.

This leads up to another case of euthanasia of inconvenience. Paso Fino horses are from Puerto Rico. They are a smallish horse that instead of the trot they perform a 'single foot' type of motion that requires no posting. The rider travels smoothly with none of the up and down of the regular trot. My client had a small but nice stable of Passo Finos with a stallion and two mares, one of which had recently foaled. The foal grew and soon caused a shortage of stalls. The foal's dam became surplus and no longer fit into the owner's plans. Realizing her diminished role in the stable, she became fretful and began to lose weight. The owner refused to give her away for fear she would be badly treated. The situation of a misfit mare in the stable began to prey on the owner's mind. The indecision about what to do with her was causing him worry and loss of sleep. He finally made the agonizing decision to put her down. He called me to make the appointment. He called me to postpone it. He called me to remake the appoint. His guilt feeling about the plans were wearing him down and affecting his well being. He became very irritable and concerned about what his neighbors might think. He called me again and this time he had reached the point of actually digging a grave for the mare which he wanted me to inspect for suitability. We again made a date. My daughter went with me for the sad moral dilemma type of euthanasia. She has great empathy with the species horse and unbeknown to us her mind was actively searching for a way out of the dilemma. The thought of leading a healthy mare to its grave was as disturbing and tragic to her as it was to the owner and me.

Nevertheless the mare was led to the site and while standing next to her grave was given a tranquilizer. I was preparing to give the fatal intravenous injection when I heard my daughter yell – "Wait! – Why don't you give me a chance to place her." The owner clearly shaken and upset with the delay said, "I'm afraid she'll be abused." "Let me try, I know a lot of horse people who might be interested and should be able to handle her difficult behavior. Give me a week." The owner wavered, not wanting to deter now that we had got this far with the dreadful job. We realized how shaken and distraught he was so we made a firm grave side compact. We all agreed that at the end of a week if she had no place for the mare to go, we would go ahead with the task without any further deliberation. The plan was set, the date was set. Done!. – We shook hands. The grave stayed empty. The owner got a good night's sleep. The mare slept in her stall and I escaped from a moral dilemma. My daughter having effected a stay of execution, went to work with a sense of urgency due the time constraint in our compact. Her memory bank contained a nucleus of many horse people from years on

the show ring and years of riding with me on veterinary calls. Many phone calls were made in which she patiently explained the situation to each. Her time limit was nearly gone. She posted a notice in the local grain store. It brought a reply. It was a woman horse client out of the past. She was interested. She met us at the owner's stable. Her child had grown into a young woman and had become a horseperson like her mother. She was eager to take the mare. A small fee was charged to validate the transfer. We were all relieved and hopeful for the mare's future.
– Done!

The mare found a new home. The owner's feeling of guilt was turned into relief. The vet was spared the burden of a moral dilemma. The daughter, turned life saving horse broker, renewed old friendships and ingratiated a troubled owner who looked forward to filling in an empty grave. We all went homeward feeling fulfilled for the day.

The ability to perform euthanasia is unique to doctors of Veterinary Medicine. Whether done as a privilege or an obligation or a moral dilemma it should be done humanely avoiding pain, anxiety and fear as much as possible.

IT ALL WASHES OFF

It's a good thing it all washes off. The phone rang and the day's schedule was scuttled. Early morning phone calls are apt to do that. It was a call for help from an elderly teacher who lived with her twin sister on a small farm a short distance from the school where they both taught. They kept two cows, partly for a hobby and partly to supply themselves and their neighbors with clean raw milk. They were known as the Boardman sisters. They were dignified, cultured, and well respected throughout the area. But this morning they were in a panic. "Besse calved during the night she has cast her wethers and she can't get up. Can you come?"

'Cast Wethers' is common language, for a prolapsed uterus. It is a classic veterinary emergency. The uterine contractions normally cease after delivery of the calf and placenta. In this case the uterus abnormally follows the new born into the birth canal where its presence stimulates continued contractions causing the uterus to invert (turn inside out) and be exteriorized. The placenta is the extraordinary membrane that mammals have that transmits nutrition by osmosis from the mother's blood to the placental blood and hence through the umbilical cord to the fetus. The mal positioned uterus soon swells and of course becomes severely contaminated.

This was Bessie's condition on this morning that brought the phone call from the distraught teachers, and disrupted my plans for the morning. And this was the scene I saw when I arrived at the barn, a life threatening emergency. The longer the delay, the more difficult the repair.

In a case like this the first procedure is to inject a local anesthesia into the base of the spine to prevent further contractions. Then the organ is cleaned and any remaining placental tissues are removed. The uterus is next gradually worked back into its normal position. The procedure is difficult and care wast be taken not to rupture the tissues. At any moment in the procedure the uterus is apt to slither out to its original mal position, losing all that has been gained. After returning it to the abdominal cavity it becomes necessary to keep it there until it shrinks to the point that further contractions will not affect it. To hold it in place a long rod with a rounded knob on the end is inserted. Careful pressure on this helps to reinvert the organ and stabilize it in its normal relationships. An injection (posterior pituitary) is given to hasten the shrinking of the uterus. Heavy sutures across the vaginal opening help prevent recurrence. All this is time consuming, exhausting and fraught with failure.

In this case on this morning the patient was unable to rise. This meant that in order to do the procedure I had to get down to her level which was the barn gutter. This I did and soon came to resemble the gutter. The whole picture was complicated by the fact that I was due at a cocktail party that afternoon. Fortunately after the cow was put back in order, she was able to rise and she started to eat. Getting up and eating are two beautiful signs of recovery. All that remained was to administer antibiotics and return in three days to remove the sutures.

I made the party smelling like a rose; the elderly teachers taught; the cow nursed her calf and the hostess of the party never realized that I had spent the morning in a gutter. This goes to show that no matter how dirty the veterinary job may be, it all washes off and one can become socially acceptable again.

CASEY IS MISSING

"I can't find Casey!" I didn't have to ask who was calling, I knew who it was and I knew he was upset. It was our friend Roy on the phone. Casey was his Morgan gelding who had been a member of his family for many years. He was ridden by Roy's daughters at horse shows, he was great on trail rides and well known for pulling a doctor's buggy in parades and most of all Casey had functioned in many weddings proudly delivering the newlyweds to their receptions. Then there was the time when Roy and I were returning from a parade with our horses and buggies. Roy's was a doctor's buggy and of course Casey was pulling it. Mine was an open buggy made out of a natural Curly Maple finish. It was pulled by our Morgan mare called Winnie. Doctor's buggies have a little oval window in the side curtain. It was through this oval window after the parade that I saw Roy's face with an ugly grin on it. I interpreted it as a challenge to race. Challenge or not, I accepted it. I let up on Winnie's reins a bit and she responded eagerly, having been held to a walk for a long time in the parade. The trip quickly degenerated into a race up Main Street Hill with a spark making trot, neck and neck straight through a red light. We had both seen the buggy race portrayed in the movie 'Friendly Persuasion' in which two neighbors raced their buggies on the way to church, and were no doubt influenced by it. I of course was Gary Cooper. To this day Jay thinks he and Casey won the race. He doesn't know that I pulled up a bit on Winnie at the end. But that's OK with me. Like I said, Casey was an important member of family and community, and he deserved to win. But tonight he was lost.

It was a cold snowy winter night when Roy's anxious phone call took me away from the fire. He went on, "Casey always goes in the wood lot and returns at feeding time. Tonight he didn't come back. I've been walking the woods for hours looking for him. He's prone to colic and he could have become sick and fallen into one of the gullies. It's snowing and he may not last long and I'm exhausted." "OK," I said, "I'll grab a coat and we'll walk the woods again." As I was leaving, it occurred to me that I should let someone know where I was going, so I called my daughter. "I'm going to help Roy find his horse, he's missing and Roy is frantic." My daughter's response was more or less what I expected. "Wait for me, I'll go with you." There was a long pause, - then,- "Dad, was he wearing a blanket?" "Never mind about a blanket," I said impatiently. "They need help and Roy is afraid Casey could be cast and dying out there." "But if he had a blanket," she yelled, "I know where he is and he is very much alive." "Yes, I think he was wearing a blanket, so where is he, and how come you know so much." "The police called me this morning," she said, "they wanted to know if I was missing a horse wearing a blanket. They said that a man had reported that a horse had wandered into his barn yard. So he put the horse into a stall and called them. It wasn't my horse," She said, "so I forgot about it. That's Roy's horse!"

I made a very sweet call to Roy with the news. We met him at the stable that was harboring his Casey. Roy was tired, tight lipped and confused that his beloved horse had left home for another stable. He just picked up his run away horse and left. Not a word was spoken. He didn't thank us. He didn't need to, we knew how he felt. We last saw him and Casey in a light snow fall silhouetted against a street light walking dejectedly homeward. We looked at each other, smiled and also went homeward, feeling fulfilled for the day.

GREAT BLUE HERON

"Dad!!" the phone interrupted my noon nap "I have a Great Blue Heron in my mud room. He's unconscious, he may be dead, you're a vet – do something!"

I had no idea what on earth to do, but I was familiar with her tone of voice which meant action – man!

It had happened like this – Nancy was looking out her kitchen window with a view down a long steep hill to a pond adjacent to the woods. This window often functioned as a virtual wild life blind. Through it she could watch all sorts of nature activities without being noticed. Through this blind she often watched fawns cavort happily around their mothers. Recently she had seen a fox approach a flock of grazing Canadian Geese in the pasture. Instead of making a panicy flight to the pond, the Geese circled their wagons with beaks pointing outward, making a formidable defense against any would be predator. The Fox left probably thinking mice would be less trouble. At other times she could watch an Otter repeatedly dive under the edge of the pond ice to return with a fish for a meal on shore. Occasionally a Coyote would appear against the woods in the evening sun. Small birds appeared according to the season and her bird feeder was a constant birding experience. Great Blue Herons frequently stood in statuesque silence in the pond's shallow water until an unsuspecting fish came within reach and then lightening strike for a meal.

This day was different. She saw a Great Blue Heron tangled in a wire, prostrate and half immersed in the water. Nancy being Nancy, set out on a rescue mission. Her dog, sensing excitement, galloped along beside her. They found the poor bird immobile, helpless, exhausted and half drowned. Her dog insisted on helping to untangle the bird but it quickly became obvious that he was more interested in predation than rescue. In order to save the victim from more injury and pressed by the urgency of the situation, Nancy warded off the dog with what could be described as a three point kick. The kickee got the message but the kicker lost a shoe in the act. The rescue mission then started to struggle up the hill. The dog bounced along bursting with excitement but staying clear of the chance of another swift kick. Nancy with one shoe off, over wet and rocky lands, bird in arms, long neck hanging one way, long legs and wings hanging in various other ways, finally gained the top. All told they made a most unusual sight.

The comatose Heron was placed in her mud room and her phone call brought me shortly to the scene. I saw the heron partly revived, and half standing on his long skinny legs, having accomplished this without benefit of any of my veterinary wisdom. Nancy was eager to tell me that while she was peeking through a window at her victim turned captive he had struck the window directly in front of what to him was a shiny object, but to her was her right eye. Heron had apparently forgotten that she had just recently saved his life. This put Nancy in a cautious mode as far as the reviving Heron was concerned. GB Heron next showed his disgust with us by disgorging a Bass out of his crop on to the floor that appeared to be much too big for his thin neck. GB Heron continued to recover until it was time to make a decision as to what to do with him. Nancy said, "Let's ease him out the door," while she handed me a broom and found safety at a distance. As I cautiously broomed GB Heron toward the door I was attacked in bayonet fashion. He made a threatening bark like noise at the same time, to emphasize his point. Nevertheless GB Heron advanced toward the door while regaining his composure, dignity and beauty. He stepped out on to the porch, he looked to the left and to the right then took flight effortlessly on great graceful wings. He understandably didn't head back to the pond. Nancy and I exchanged glances, proud of our effort and amazed at the result. I said, "Are you going to cook the fish." She said, "Go home." Which I did to finish my nap.

PART OF THE SOLUTION

"You last client has a Dachshund that needs to be neutered." "OK," I said, "I'm expecting them, send them in." The dog was entered and I sensed that the owner was eager to talk. I knew he was involved with Animal Welfare so I was eager to listen. We repaired to the kitchen for coffee, he talked and I listened. He started by explaining what he called the 'un-' dogs. Too many puppies are unplanned, unwanted, unfortunate, unhealthy, unhappy and unloved. How to remove the 'un' prefix he admitted was complex but neutering was an important part of the solution. Which is what brought him and his dog to my hospital.

Since I appeared to be a willing listener, he told me his 'part of the solution' story.

He went on – "Our biological clock had run out long ago. Nevertheless my wife and I had a late in life baby. It's true that most people would recognize the baby as a Dachshund puppy. But they obviously had poor vision or poor imagination. Our baby came to us minus the 'un' prefix. He was planned, healthy and happy. I mentioned one day to my wife that it was too bad that our baby had crooked front legs. She fired back, "That comes from your side of the family." This was dangerous territory, so I dropped it and left the scene muttering about how my legs were perfectly straight."

He went on – "We called our baby, 'Dot Com' and he grew and played and gave us much joy. Generally Dot Com was very bright but he was slow to learn how to lift his leg onto bushes, tires and such. He was so late with that skill that when he finally performed the act, we all cheered. He didn't understand what the excitement was all about but the attention pleased him."

Not long after that my wife admonished me that Dot could possibly become a cause of some 'un' puppies. It was time I had a father son talk with him. Not having done that for many decades, I approached him with trepidation. "Dot my boy," I said, "Come sit, I want your attention for awhile. You are at an age when you are going to sense a new attraction for the girl dogs. It will be very difficult for you to resist doing a wrong thing and ruining a young girl's life. You must be patient and act like a gentleman. Dot Com – <u>please pay attention</u> and get your mind off my bowl of clam chowder." Our late in life child looked at me with pity. "Pop, I've know that stuff for a long time, stop sweating, I promise not to chase the girls, cool it, I promise, I promise. Is there a Bible in the house?"

When my wife appeared, I proudly related my accomplishment at having done my fatherly duty. "I'm sure he will be an example of decorum, the envy of the neighborhood. He promised, he even asked for a Bible."

"Promises, promises – he shortly became a eunich. It must have been her side of the family.

Whereupon Dot Com became part of he solution and grew to be a leader among his people.

As I said, DotCom's father wanted to talk and I wanted to listen, which we both did.

PETER'S COAST GUARD RECRUIT

Peter had thirty years of hard luck with dogs. Thirty years of unhealthy dogs. He was a devoted owner and he nurtured them throughout their lives regardless.

His first dog was a Shepherd type who early on developed a weakness in his jaw muscles. It was an auto immune type of disorder in which his immune system attacked the jaw muscles on top of his head. His dog learned to live with the handicap, but he drooled. He drooled all the time, he drooled for ten years. Amazingly Peter's next dog developed a muscle weakness all over that required ten years of pills to keep him up right. Peter was faithful and unrelenting in his commitment to his dogs. The third dog was a Rottweiller that grew to be over one hundred pounds and had an attitude like a junk yard dog. He was very intolerant of strangers and remarkably intolerant of vets. Peter put up with the dog's attitude for many years until one time. – A visiting friend claiming he knew all about dogs, attempted to befriend the Rottweiller. Beer in hand he approached the dog on the safe side of his fence. He put his face up close to the fence and made friendly cooing sounds. This gesture of truce failed and the dog hit the fence so hard that the guy fell over backward, spilling his beer on himself. Peter regretfully decided to divest himself of his angry charge.

The US Coast Guard at this time was asking for donations of dogs suitable for guard duty. Peter volunteered his dog. He was sent a list of health exams to be checked out by a vet as a condition of acceptance. This brought the two of them to my office. There was a long list of required examinations. With trepidation I proceeded. Peter and the dog were about the same weight but hardly the same strength. Peter's attempt at restraint found him sliding around on the floor trying desperately to keep the dog from eating me as I made the examinations. We succeeded in covering the heart, lungs, temperature, ears, eyes, skin, teeth and locomotion, and found them normal. Eventually I came to the last request for an examination and it brought me up short. It was 'check the tonsils'. I considered asking him to stick his tongue out so I could use a tongue depressor to view them, but scuttled the idea. My devotion to duty went south at that point and I put down 'tonsils unavailable due to aggressive dentition.' So Peter's Rotweller and his elusive tonsils joined the Coast Guard and found good use for his bad attitude. Peter's fourth dog was perfect and therefore not of a nature worth mentioning. A life time of good dog news fails to add to the story.

LADY BUG

My respect for the Lady Bug was enhanced lately when I read that the pretty little turtle like bug with spots is a natural enemy of the Wooly Adelgrid, an aphid which destroys many of our Hemlock Trees. My respect for the Lady Bug was increased again when a young lad came into the office with his mother and the family cat. The boy was very carefully carrying a small box under his arm. When I asked him what was in the box he obliged me by showing his treasure. It was a lady Bug named Spotty. I was pleased with the boy's taste in pets but glad that it didn't need any treatment from me.

Since most of the time was used up by Spotty, the family cat got rather quickly dealt with. Who can compete with a Lady Bug?

AT THE FARMER'S FAIR

It was at a farmers' yearly gathering where the farmers remind folks of what they contribute to our tables with their locally grown produce. It was pure Americana. I admired the farmers and their produce, but what really caught my attention was some ex farmer clients out of the past. As I ambled down the row of exhibits I approached a couple with wide smiles on their faces. When I got into my ever decreasing range of eye focus, I recognized an old fellow bee keeper client. That was fun and we reminisced about how we had captured a large swarm of bees. The swarm was near a restaurant and was driving customers away. He then told us how he has to medicate his hives against infections and mites in order to keep them productive. That made me glad that I was long out of the honey bee hobby. I ambled on past the exhibits of the apple growers, pear growers and other food producers. I looked at wonderful new tractors and equally wonderful old and older tractors. Then I ran into another native who looked familiar but I couldn't recognize him until he explained that I had doctored his father's cows when he was a small boy. This activated his memory and he was eager to retell a story. Memories are so all prevailing at my age that I sometimes try to blank them out in order to make room for thoughts about the now and the future. But this was a day for memories. Anyhow, after each of us exaggerated our answer to the customary, 'How are you,' greeting, he began to talk, and then the fun began.

He asked me if I remembered calling his father and brother Matt Dillon and Chester. I wavered a bit in my response so he grabbed at the chance to tell the story. His story went like this. Their farm was on a hill overlooking their saw mill yard some distance away at the bottom of the hill. On the night of his story they had noticed tail lights of a truck down in their lumber yard. There had been boards missing lately from the yard, so my father was filled with rightful indignation and was becoming trigger happy in that regard. He immediately grabbed his double barreled shot gun off the rack and my younger brother Harley away from watching 'Gun Smoke' on the television. With the attitude of a sheriff and his deputy they marched down the hill toward the lumber yard. Harley bounced along happily anticipating his role as a deputy. As they approached the entrance to the lumber yard and saw the thievery going on, my father's indignation increased and he broke into a trot. That exertion caused the gun to go off barely missing Harley who immediately lost all interest in being a deputy and started back up the hill. My father quickly collared the deserter and forced him to rejoin the ranks. At any rate the explosion forewarned the thieves who jumped into their truck intent on escape. But my father had other intentions. As the truck met him making its exit from the yard, he bayoneted the shot gun through the truck window directly into the face of the thieving driver and commanded him to halt and get out. Having already heard a shot the thieves knew my father wasn't bashful about firing the gun and since the barrel was now inches from his head, it quickly occurred to the driver that discretion was the better part of escape. They complied and exited the truck without complication. Of course they had no way of knowing that there had been only one shell in the gun and that was gone in the first volley. The thieves were then marched up the hill with a shot gun at their collective behinds. Harley was again enjoying his role as deputy and was jumping up and down with excitement. Back at the farm my father, by this time enjoying his role as a sheriff, became downright mean. He ordered the captives to hit the ground while his deputy ran in to call the local police. You can see my father was very resentful about his missing lumber. The police were glad to be involved with a real live crime and responded smartly. They were of course shocked to see two alleged crooks held on the ground at gun point and quickly rescued them by dispatching them into the cruiser. Then the police had some discussion as to whether or not to arrest my father for assault with a dangerous weapon when they should have been called in the first place.

My father was not arrested and the would be thieves were released because my father refused to press charges. I think he figured that henceforth they would likely lose interest in his lumber yard and they might spread the word about the difficulties of pilfering from it, which was really all my father wanted.

That is the way it was on that night when my friend's father took the law into his own hands. And that is why I had called his father and brother Matt Dillon and Chester and that is why it all came back to me at the farmers' fair.

CONTENTMENT

Communication across species is always remarkable. Perhaps the best example of it is a dog taking verbal orders from its trainer, or a dressage horse exquisitely taking aids from the rider. On the Serengeti of Africa Wildebeest graze in peace while a Lion rests near by. The moment the Lion displays a predatory mode the relationship changes. The message becomes, "I intend to eat you." It is an obvious and every day cross species communication experience for many species. On the other hand, communication displays of contentment are what this little piece is about. Top on the familiar list of cross species contentment communication has to be the ubiquitous tail wag of dogs which many times elevates to expression of joy. The purring of a cat is a unique and common cross species contentment communication. I had a crow once who would sit beside me on the lawn and make a low contented noise. Visit a dairy barn and look at the expression on the face a cow chewing her cud. You will see a display of contentment hard to match.

But this contentment subject is brought up because of a rare cross species communication that I became familiar with. It was a habit my Standard Bred mare developed. She was a constant companion of mine either on trail rides or in family polo games. She had an agreeable and consistent habit of making a welcome noise when I approached her stall. This could be described as a nasal flutter. She did this by contracting her little false nostrils, and she would do this every time I approached her. Strangers in the barn often expressed concern that my mare had a 'heavey' type breathing. (Heaves is a severe type of emphysema). They were often hard to convince that it was an elective noise. But I knew she meant it as a way of telling me she was pleased that I was there. It was a cross species display of contentment that appeared to be unique between us. At times she let folks think she had 'heaves' to take advantage of the sympathy she might get.

COMPASSION VS CASH

As I have said before, a coffee break at the diner can generate unexpected tales and information. This morning I was joined by the local Dog Officer whom I have known for a long time. She has succeeded in carrying out her job for years and increased the efficiency of it by incorporating computered information on all the dogs. The result is that a stray dog is as rare as a Coyote about town. She was upset this morning and wanted to talk. I was willing to listen so it went like this.

She said an elderly woman called her in great distress because her ancient cat was under her bed crying in pain. The cat had been in failing health for some time and she realized it was time to deliver her from her pain. The Dog Officer asked if she had called her vet. Yes she had, but the office had asked for the money in advance and more for disposal of the body. The owner had agreed but would they wait until her Social Security check came. "No", was the answer. My officer friend then asked, "Are you a client of this practice?" "Yes," the owner said. "Do you owe them any money?" "No," the owner said. "They refused to help me without the money." My friend, being the kind of person she is took matters into her own hands. She did not want the senior lady and the cat to suffer needlessly and often acted over and above the call of duty. She gathered up the cat and presented it to the vet herself. The cat was put down and paid for by the Dog Officer who was paid back shortly afterward out of the owner's next check.

I suggested to her that the character of a professional person is well formed long before he becomes a professional and learning a profession does not assure a sense of compassion or empathy along with the degree. I went on, "The preface of my little book speaks of not wanting the old fashioned vets to pass without being noticed. A sad story like yours hopefully isn't typical, but begs for some of the old values and some of your compassionate values to find a place in the character of a person before becoming professional.

We both agreed, finished our coffee and went on our way.

About the Author

Shortly after graduating from college in 1942 I found myself interning in a general practice. I was soon delegated to the large animals because I hadn't developed a bedside manner to suit the small animal owners. This meant that dairy cows and draft horses benefited from my efforts. It was hard work but had the advantage of giving me deferment from the service. The companion horse had not reached its present popularity at that time. The draft horses were being used for deliveries as a substitute for trucks due to Wartime gas rationing. After two years I went on my own and lost my deferment rating. After time in the service I started again in a small town in South Central Massachusetts. They had been without a veterinarian for years so I was generally well received. In the normal chronology of things our family eventually consisted of a boy and three girls. We were living a nearly normal life when a gift horse dramatically changed it. The horse exposed the native empathy and talent our daughters had with the equine. This started a long evolution of a farm, more horses, an indoor arena, many horse shows, eventually giving lessons in saddle and hunt seat and bringing home a Morgan Horse Grand National Award from Oklahoma City. As I look back I think the gift horse set up a life style that helped us raise four children free of serious problems. They all had responsibilities with their horses that were more important to them than the dangerous temptations so many of our young are exposed to. I'm glad I didn't look that gift horse in the mouth.

CPSIA information can be obtained at www.ICGtesting.com
Printed in the USA
BVOW020427240912

301137BV00001B/1/A